DOWN'S SYNDROME

Past, Present and Future

Dr BRIAN STRATFORD

Penguin Books

PENGUIN BOOKS

Published by the Penguin Group
Penguin Books Ltd, 27 Wrights Lane, London W8 5TZ, England
Penguin Books USA Inc., 375 Hudson Street, New York, New York 10014, USA
Penguin Books Australia Ltd, Ringwood, Victoria, Australia
Penguin Books Canada Ltd, 10 Alcorn Avenue, Toronto, Ontario, Canada M4V 3B2
Penguin Books (NZ) Ltd, 182–190 Wairau Road, Auckland 10, New Zealand

Penguin Books Ltd, Registered Offices: Harmondsworth, Middlesex, England

First published 1989
10 9 8 7 6 5 4 3

Printed in England by Clays Ltd, St Ives plc
Filmset in Monophoto Sabon

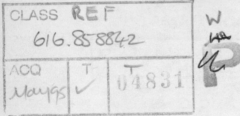

For Philippa Julia
and Mark Richard John

CONTENTS

ACKNOWLEDGEMENTS

I owe so much to so many people that it would be impossible to name them all, especially all the people with Down's syndrome in many parts of the world who make my work such a pleasure. Also I must thank their parents and guardians who provide such an inspiration.

I want to thank a number of people who have been particularly helpful to me in writing this book. I will not be so formal as to name them alphabetically but will confess my gratitude as I recall them, so the order of acknowledgement has no particular importance.

The first Vice-Chancellor of the University of Nottingham, Dr Bertrand Hallward, now living in retirement in Cambridge, talked to me about the Greeks; Dr Horace Thuline first drew my attention to the Olmecs; Emeritus Professor Robert Markus translated the passages from the writings of St Augustine; Dr Marie Cerna and Hana Svobodova of Czechoslovakia searched for the history of the paintings at the Castle Hradec, and Professor Voci, Emeritus Professor Alistair Smart and Dr Michael Kidd combined to authenticate my interest in the paintings of Mantegna.

Professor Joe Berg was extremely cooperative on the subject of radiation and his collaborator Dr George Smith was helpful in many ways, not least of which was to find for me an obscure academic thesis concerning the dwellers in Ancient Mexico. My confidence in various controversial issues in Down's syndrome is always strengthened by Dr Sigfried Pueschel and the quiet assurance of Dr John Rynders. I am also extremely grateful for and honoured by the generous help I always receive from Professor Jerome Lejeune.

My research associate Jonathan Steele is consistently dependable and has the ability to describe highly complicated biological processes in simple language. I owe Jonathan a great deal.

Though not *directly* involved in the book, there are those friends who have shaped and modified my views and have, through their conversations, had more influence than they know: Emeritus Professor E. A. Lunzer, Professor Peter Mittler, Emeritus Professor J. F. Eggleston, Dr Cliff Cunningham, Professor Jean Rondal, Sir Brian Rix, Professor Stanley Segal, Dr Victor Shields, Professor Gwynn Roberts, Dr Georgio Albertini, Mtra Sylvia Escamilla, Professor Paolo Meazzini, Professor Kenneth Holt, Dr Pat Gunn, Professor Campbell Murdoch, Professor Ishwar Verma, Dr Rene Eminyan, Professor Reuven Feuerstein, Dr Manny Chigier, Henning Hansmann, the late Dr Thomas Weihs; there are many others who I hope will forgive me if I have not recorded their names – my gratitude does not go unrecorded.

My many friends, colleagues and former students in Hong Kong deserve a special mention, but especially those closely connected with my work in Down's syndrome: Evonne Ching, David Ip, Jonathan Chamberlain and Carmen Au. Students are always a source of help and inspiration to a university lecturer and I could not name all the students who have been helpful in these ways, though I must mention Howard Byers and Sue Weeden; and Nick Crawford of Hong Kong University. I appreciate also the loyal support I always receive from the Director and staff, Chairman and Executive Committee of the Down's Syndrome Association in Britain.

Special thanks go to my secretary Jill Cleaver, who is one of the very few people who can decipher my handwriting, and to Deborah Watchorn of Southern Television, for producing the graphics. I would also like to thank Pam Dix of Penguin Books who has kept me going, been enthusiastic and been more than helpful in her constructive criticisms and suggestions.

The final word must go to my wife Maureen, who has not only kept my scientific language under reasonable control but has been positively helpful in a thousand other ways. Any credit for this book must go to her and to all those I have mentioned above; the faults are entirely mine.

BRIAN STRATFORD
Nottingham 1988

INTRODUCTION

This book is *about* Down's syndrome. It tells the story of Down's syndrome and the attitudes people have held in past times to the mentally handicapped in general and to Down's syndrome in particular. It outlines the mistakes which have been made as well as the discoveries which have led to our present understanding of the condition.

Scientific discoveries sometimes require scientific language to describe them. Where this is inevitable, the principles have been explained in a manner which it is hoped is accessible to the non-scientific reader. For example, it would not be possible to tell the full story of Down's syndrome without some explanation of its biological basis, though this aspect has been placed in an Appendix (page 156), to be turned to when, and if, such information is required. The human story has taken precedence over the scientific.

Facts have not been distorted to suit personal opinion, but personal opinions, while kept to a minimum, have not been avoided. The book is intended for the general reader as well as for parents, and they too will have their opinions. Hopefully the book will stimulate debate. As this is not a text book it does not attempt an exhaustive survey of research findings; such information is available from a range of literature in the field of mental handicap. This also means that the sources of evidence for some statements are not always included, though reliable sources have always been consulted.

The story begins with the Olmecs of ancient Mexico, the first culture to have left artefacts which represent Down's syndrome, though the absolute beginning of Down's syndrome would be with Genesis, the creation of human life, and would begin when people started to multiply. Down's syndrome is therefore not a disease, it is part of our rich and varied biological inheritance.

It would, however, be totally unrealistic to suggest that children with Down's syndrome cause no problems; of course they do. To begin with, it is difficult for parents to come to terms with the birth of such a child. Certainly unexpected and major adjustments have to be made, and these adjustments have to be made without experience or an adequate model to help; but the majority of parents of children with Down's syndrome sooner or later learn to accommodate to the new situation and actually enjoy life with their child. The real problems are not with the child, nor are they with the parents or with other members of the family. It is the so-called normal community, with its lack of understanding, that can make life difficult.

How then might we take a fresh view of the handicapped child?

Suppose we were to ask Rubinstein to play Chopin on an out-of-tune piano with some of the keys missing. Would we conclude from the resulting sound that Rubinstein was a poor pianist? Of course not; we would recognize that he had been given an inadequate and imperfect instrument to play on.

The late Dr Thomas Weihs used to ask the question: 'Who do I say "I" to when I say "I" to myself?' It cannot be said that we say 'I' to our bodies. We are rarely really satisfied with our bodies, they are either too fat or too thin or too lazy – we are never totally at one with our bodies. Our bodies are constantly undergoing change, but the 'I' that I said to myself twenty years ago refers to the same me. We do not love someone less if they lose an arm and we do not love a fat man more because there is more of him. Do we then say 'I' to our thoughts? This cannot be so either, because I am often ashamed of my thoughts, if they are of anger or jealousy or resentment. Who then is ashamed? If we think carefully about this concept we will realize that the 'I' of the most seriously handicapped child is as perfect as our own. It might then be concluded that a child is not handicapped within the scope of the child's existence, that child is only handicapped in relation to the kind of demands which are made by the society in which he or she lives, and the same applies to their parents, relations and friends. It is hoped that this book might make a few more friends for those who are 'handicapped' by Down's syndrome.

BRIAN STRATFORD

CHAPTER 1

WHAT IS DOWN'S SYNDROME?

There is a story about a medical student who was taking his final oral examination and was answering all the questions very well indeed; he knew he was doing well. The professor was impressed and was almost finished. Then he said, 'Just one final question, Mr Johnson. What is the cause of Down's syndrome?' The question worried the student because he did not want to end the examination in an unsatisfactory way. He hesitated and then answered, 'I'm sorry, professor, I *did* know but I have forgotten.' The professor looked at the student sadly and said, 'That's a great pity, Mr Johnson, because now nobody knows.'

The primary cause of Down's syndrome still remains one of the unsolved mysteries of human genetics. However, the mechanism by which it happens is well understood. When cells begin to divide at conception, some of the thread-like bodies inside the cells, called *chromosomes*, do not divide as they should. This 'error' is called *non-disjunction*. Why that should happen so regularly in the human race is unknown.

Down's syndrome, formerly called 'mongolism' when it was first isolated from other mentally disabling conditions, is the most common form of severe mental retardation. It accounts for about one third of all seriously mentally handicapped people, though not all people with Down's syndrome are severely mentally handicapped. There are some individuals whose intelligence is within the normal range and quite a number who could be described as only mildly handicapped. Yet they all have in common that slightly oriental appearance which gave rise to the first descriptive label, 'mongol'. Anyone who knows children with Down's syndrome well will agree that they resemble their parents more than they resemble each other, though it cannot be denied that the child with

Down's syndrome is easily recognizable by a distinctively character-istic appearance. That is perhaps unfortunate, because it singles them out and tends to give a popular impression that they must be all the same, with the same degree of mental retardation. This distinctive appearance has another unfortunate consequence which is that it signals 'mental deficiency'; a kind of archetype which represents all those hidden 'ancestral' fears associated with 'mental' disturbances.

An interesting fact concerning those physical features of Down's syndrome with which we are so familiar is that all children with Down's syndrome do not have all the classical signs, or *stigmata* as scientists prefer to call them. Usually it is obvious; there can be no mistaking that the person we see has Down's syndrome. Sometimes we need to look twice and even then there may be some doubt. It is natural for us to declare that those with fewer *stigmata* will be less affected than those whose *stigmata* make their condition clear. This is not so. The same deduction has been of sufficient interest for a number of studies to have been conducted on this question. Results have shown that number of *stigmata* is not related to in-tellectual or social functioning. In other words, those people with Down's syndrome who look less obviously like the 'archetype' may not be the most intelligent of the Down's syndrome population, and those whose appearance leaves no doubt that they are people with Down's syndrome may be 'brighter than they look'. This is not so strange when we transfer this same concept to the so-called normal population: how many people who are very bright indeed look dull, and how many who look highly intelligent are in-tellectually below average? This is a fact which is important for parents to bear in mind.

Before the discovery was made that Down's syndrome had a particular and unique *genetic* characteristic which could be ex-amined under a microscope, leaving no doubt as to the diagnosis, the diagnosis had to be made by adding up the *stigmata* and then carefully watching subsequent development. This explains why, in the past, some children with Down's syndrome were not finally diagnosed until the age of 2 or 3, or even later.

Incidence and prevalence

Apart from occasional environmental influences, the rate of conception of Down's syndrome infants has not changed dramatically through the ages. The incidence rate also seems to have remained unchanged, at one in 600–700 live births. This incidence rate is universal and is not influenced by race, colour, culture or climate. Prevalence, however, is another matter. Prevalence refers to those people with Down's syndrome who survive and grow up in a community, and obviously then, prevalence is influenced by a number of environmental factors. These factors would include:

1. The effect of better health care.
2. The effect of change of average maternal child-bearing age.
3. The possibility of under-diagnosis.
4. The effect of pre-natal diagnosis.

Better health care

Improving health care over the years has had the effect of increasing the prevalence of Down's syndrome, through extending life expectancy and also increasing the likelihood of survival of an affected foetus. It would be reasonable to speculate that further medical advances could reduce certain specific problems associated with Down's syndrome (such as cardiac and respiratory problems and the onset of Alzheimer's disease) and consequently create a further rise in the Down's syndrome population. These issues will be discussed in greater detail later.

Maternal child-bearing age

The effect of maternal age on the birth incidence of Down's syndrome is well known and well documented, being first mentioned by Frazer and Mitchell in a paper published in 1876. Various theories have been put forward to account for this age effect. The question of the time ova are held 'in suspense' in the female is a factor which must be taken into account (see page 163). It has also been suggested in the medical literature that changes in hormones might be involved, because hormones certainly influence maturation

Table 1. Cumulative rates of Down's syndrome per 1,000 live births in older women [From a paper by E. B. Hook (1982)].

Maternal age (year)	New York	Sweden	Massachussetts
All ≥ 30	3.39	3.19	3.15
All ≥ 35	6.61	6.68	5.96
All ≥ 40	14.48	17.70	14.20
All ≥ 45	38.40	62.09	35.25

of ova. There would therefore tend to be an increased risk of chromosomal problems as women approach the end of their child-bearing years. The hormones are also connected with other factors associated with age and these are not always related to *older* mothers. There is, for example, an increased risk to very young mothers which might be connected with immature hormone control.

It must be remembered also that the majority of children with Down's syndrome are born to mothers aged between 20 and 29 years. This of course is because the majority of all children are born to mothers in this age range. Table 1 gives some idea of the greater risk in older women. Hook tabulated the maternal age effect from three of his studies in different areas. He considered that the mean maternal child-bearing age has decreased in Europe and America and notes that this is reflected in the birth incidence[1] of Down's syndrome in many European and American studies, which he reports to have dropped from 1.5 per 1,000 in the 1950s to 1.0-1.2 per 1,000 in the 1970s.

There is also some speculation which suggests that the contraceptive pill may be associated with an increase in the number of children with Down's syndrome born to younger mothers. This speculation has important implications and will be discussed more fully later.

A word should be included here about paternal age. Until recently the age of fathers was considered to be of no significance, but more recent studies have called this 'fact' into question. The conclusion

1. Incidence is defined as the ratio of affected live births to the total number of live births in a population. Prevalence refers to the number of living persons with Down's syndrome per 10,000 of a specified total population.

drawn from a series of investigations is that there is a significantly increased risk for fathers over the age of 55 years. However, I understand from Professor J. M. Berg, a leading authority in genetic aspects of Down's syndrome, that he dismisses paternal influence as a serious factor.

The effects of under-diagnosis and pre-natal diagnosis

There has been discussion in the medical literature that there is probably under-diagnosis of Down's syndrome at birth which leads to an under-estimation of its prevalence. Although the question is still unresolved, it does point to the need for increased provision of clinical genetic services. The over-stretching of present services in Britain could lead to *pre-natal* under-diagnosis of Down's syndrome. Strong arguments have been put forward outlining the need for more consultants in the United Kingdom who have a special interest in neonatology. The resolving of these problems in the National Health Service in the UK would help to ease some of the pressures being put upon present neonatal services, and if this could come about, under-diagnosis could be expected to diminish. This is perhaps a question of priorities in the National Health Service.

Diagnosis at the pre-natal stage and the alternative methods will be taken up later, but it is interesting to note that the availability of therapeutic termination of pregnancy following pre-natal diagnosis does not seem to have affected birth incidence of Down's syndrome to any great extent. Indeed, a study carried out in Birmingham not so very long ago reported a Down's syndrome birth rate of 1.62 per 1,000, which is very close to the frequently quoted 1 in 660, a figure which seems to have remained constant throughout the ages; survival is another matter.

Prevalence of Down's syndrome in Britain

If special provision of any kind is to be made for people with Down's syndrome, particularly in times of financial constraint, it is essential to have a reasonable estimate of the actual number of those who will be requiring some kind of special provision, at least in such major fields as medical care, social services and education.

Table 2(a). Sheffield area: number of Down's syndrome individuals, total area population and Down's syndrome prevalence in population, by age bands (end of 1983).

Age band (year)	Number of DS cases	Total population in 1,000s*	Prevalence per 10,000
1–4†	7	22.9	3.1
5–9	21	29.7	7.1
10–14	25	40.7	6.1
15–19	37	46.3	8.0
20–24	55	46.7	11.8
25–44	106	137.8	7.7
45–64	27	138.9	1.9
65 +	2	91.1	0.2
Total	280	545.8	5.13

* These are the most recent figures available, but are for mid-1982. As the population may have increased since then, a slight over-estimate of the prevalence rate would be possible.
† This does not include births for the years 1981 and 1982. As the 1–2 year-old age group may be expected to be of reasonable size, this effect may be more than compensated for in the Total prevalence figure of 5.13 per 10,000.

Though advances are being made in the development of case registers for the mentally handicapped, the number of people with Down's syndrome at present living in Britain is not readily available. Apart from the USA, where such statistics are well kept, the situation is worse in many other countries.

My colleague Jonathan Steele and I, in an attempt to provide a reasonable estimate, made an exhaustive investigation of the number of people with Down's syndrome, in a range of age groups, in two areas of Britain. Taking Sheffield as a large industrial area and Buckinghamshire as a more rural area, we were able to make some rough statistical inferences about the population as a whole. Although the final calculations were speculative in nature, we estimated that there were, in 1985, *at least* 26,000 people with Down's syndrome residing in the United Kingdom. The results of this investigation are summarized in Table 2.

The situation is not going to get better – or worse, depending on the individual interpretation of the data – because as medical services improve, the survival of people with Down's syndrome will improve with them. The future needs to be considered at the present time, with past experiences serving as a lesson.

Table 2(b). Buckinghamshire area: number of Down's syndrome individuals, total area population and Down's syndrome prevalence in population, by age bands (end of 1983).

Age band (year)	Number of DS cases	Total population in 1,000s*		Prevalence per 10,000
1–4	33	(38.761)	40.9	8.1
5–9	32	(42.412)	44.8	7.1
10–14	38	(47.718)	50.4	7.5
15–19	47	(48.76)	51.5	9.1
20–24	25	(39.327)	41.5	6.0
25–44	50	(163.519)	172.6	2.9
45–64	25	(117.251)	123.7	2.0
65 +	0	(64.473)	68.0	0.0
Total	250	599.4†		4.2

* Figures in parentheses are taken from the 1981 census. To prevent possible over-estimation of prevalence rate, these have been adjusted as follows:

$$\text{Estimate} = \frac{\text{Total population at end 1983}}{\text{Total 1981 census population}} \times (1981 \text{ census population for band})$$

†This figure is correct at the end of 1983.

Table 2(c). Possible Down's syndrome populations, from projections of total United Kingdom populations.

Year	Total population in 10,000s*	DS rate per 10,000 (prevalence)	Estimated DS population
1981	5625.2	4.63	26,045
1991	5691.2	4.63	26,350
2001	5796.8	4.63	26,839
2011	5840.3	4.63	27,041
2021	5930.7	4.63	27,459

* Taken from Central Statistical Office (1984).

CHAPTER 2

DISCOVERY OF THE GENETIC CAUSE

Human genetics

It is by now fairly well known that there is an extra chromosome present in the genetic condition of people with Down's syndrome. Some may be aware that the extra chromosome is number 21, hence the other name by which the condition is known: trisomy 21. What this actually means may be less well understood. Obviously, to have learnt that there is an *extra* chromosome present in people with Down's syndrome, it first had to be known how many chromosomes were present in the *normal* human constitution. It may come as something of a surprise to learn that this was not finally established until the year 1956, little more than thirty years ago.

Cells and chromosomes

Cytology, the study of cells, though a relatively new science, can still be traced back to early in the last century. At that time, of course, the microscope was not so well developed as it is today; its resolution was relatively poor and techniques for its use were less sophisticated. In spite of the lack of technical developments, however, it was discovered as early as 1835 that the human body was made up of *cells* which both renewed themselves and also increased in number, this increase being achieved by the cells dividing themselves. By the middle of the nineteenth century, a number of thread-like bodies had been observed in the nuclei (the mass in the centre of the cells). From then on attempts began to be made to count how many of these 'threads' were present in each cell and to observe something about their characteristics. Towards the end of the century it was seen that these 'threads' were distinctly separate segments and they began to be referred to as 'chromosomes'. This was because by chemical staining they would take colour, making them easier to count (Gr. *chroma* = colour). At this period counting the actual number of these tiny thread-like chromosomes in each cell was by no means easy. Apart from the problems of poor microscopic resolution, chromosomes bunched, overlapped and generally eluded the skill of those attempting to count them. Each time one number was put forward as being the 'correct' number of chromosomes in the human cell, another would be claimed with equal confidence. At different times in the nineteenth century 18, 24 and even 'more than 40' were proposed.

By the turn of the century the body of scientific opinion, based on the work of a number of scientists working independently, was that there were 24 chromosomes in the nucleus of the cell of the human species. This count was not, however, accepted by all scientists, confident claims for 16, 36 and 22 coming from other researchers in the field. Then, in 1912, Winiwarters published his classic work on *spermatogenesis,* the formation of sperm. He had noted that chromosomes were diploid (i.e. paired) and his count came to 47 in males, made up of 23 pairs of similar kind and an X chromosome. In females he counted 48, including two X chromosomes. Winiwarters had come very close to the actual correct number (46), yet it was to take another forty-four years finally to resolve the issue.

The situation was almost resolved in 1921 when an investigation by Painter indicated both X and Y chromosomes to be present in males, so providing evidence that there were equal numbers of chromosomes in males and females. These sex chromosomes were named X and Y for the simple reason that their shape is that of the letters X and Y. Painter's plates showed counts between 45 and 48, but the clearest of his plates showed 46. Unfortunately, when Painter published a fuller description of his work two years later he had been too much influenced by the currently established weight of scientific evidence in favour of 48. It is interesting to speculate that had he remained confident in his earlier finding of 46 chromosomes then trisomy 21 (Down's syndrome) might well have been discovered sooner. Even so, this should not detract from Painter's important discovery of a Y chromosome in males. For the next thirty years, the human chromosome complement of 48 was broadly accepted by the scientific community.

Even in these early years of the century it was being considered that Down's syndrome might have a chromosomal origin. At least five scientists published proposals that the origin of the Down's syndrome condition lay with the chromosomes. Waardenburg, the most frequently quoted authority, suggested in 1932 that either a duplication of chromosomes or a chromosome deletion might be responsible. Bleyer hit on the true cause in 1934 but had no supporting evidence. He actually suggested that *non-disjunction* might be involved. He wrote:

There may be an unequal migration of the chromosomes to the poles of the germ cell during the reduction period, *which will result in a cell progeny having a number of chromosomes unlike the number present in the parent* [my italics].

A chromosome anomaly was also suggested by others a little later. This cause was considered by Turpin and his associates, by Penrose and by Fanconi, all working in the late 1930s. They also believed that perhaps some kind of mutation might be involved in Down's syndrome. This hypothesis still worries us today in terms of the possible effects of irradiation.

Perhaps the most important, though almost forgotten, work in this field came from a woman researcher called Mittwoch, who was painstakingly investigating the number of chromosomes present in the cells in the human species. The actual number had still not been established in the early 1950s. Mittwoch must surely be credited with coming the closest to uncovering the trisomy prior to 1959. She had studied the chromosomes in a photographic plate prepared from a biopsy, and in 1952 reported:

. . . the chromosomes were not sufficiently distinct from one another to make an exact count possible; nevertheless, the approximate number of 48 chromosomes could be made out in several cells.

Consequently, at that time she was bound to conclude that the number of chromosomes appeared to be normal.

If only she had known then that the normal diploid human chromosome number was 46 and not 48, she would no doubt have looked further. One photomicrograph reproduced in her paper shows apparently 23 autosomal pairs and the X-Y pair. Yet the vast range in size of these structures could have allowed the interpretation, at that degree of resolution, that one of these 'pairs' was in fact a single small chromosome. This being the case, Mittwoch may have been the first to observe, but not to perceive, the extra chromosome in Down's syndrome.

Some four years later, in 1956, results of observations by Tijo and Levan were published. These were to unseat the long accepted views of Painter and set the stage for the discovery of the trisomy. Using a cell-squashing technique to spread the chromosomes and carefully observing the process under the microscope to ensure that no chromosomes 'escaped', they reported:

We were surprised to find that the chromosome number of 46 predominated in the tissue cultures from all four embryos.

They then looked back and decided to reappraise some of their discarded work, carried out in the previous year on a study of liver cells. They pointed out that they had decided to abandon this work because counts of 46 rather than 48 chromosomes had been found and they had assumed that something had gone wrong with their experiments. Shortly afterwards other researchers reported repeated counts of 46 chromosomes in a number of larger-scale studies. Thus the accuracy of these counts by Tijo and Levan was confirmed. At last it was established that 46 chromosomes was the exact diploid number in the normal human cell.

Perhaps it is too easy to dismiss the work of these early scientists with brief descriptions; too easy to focus on the differences between their results, and with hindsight, too easy to criticize. Possibly the most accurate assessment of this early research was made by Ford and Hamerton, the scientists whose large-scale study had finally confirmed that there were 46 chromosomes in the cells of man. Referring to all the previous research in human cytology, they wrote in the journal *Nature:* 'The wonder is that there is so little to alter.'

Discovery of the trisomy

The discovery that there were not 48 but only 46 chromosomes in the human karyotype[1] caused a renewed interest in the study of

1 The characteristics of a set of chromosomes.

human cytogenetics. Only three years later, what was to become a historic observation was reported at the end of a short article about human chromosomes in tissue cultures. It read:

In three boys with Down's syndrome, the chromosome number found in different preparations was 47, for each of the three individuals. [Translated from Lejeune, Gauthier and Turpin(1959a)]

Seven weeks later, in March, Lejeune and his colleagues published their second famous article, this time specifically reporting the chromosome findings in nine children with Down's syndrome. They had found 47 chromosomes in most of the cells that were examined, and offered the explanation that non-disjunction between a pair of the smallest chromosomes might have occurred at meiosis (a process in cell division). However, their language was measured and they were cautious about their results. They noted that it was not yet possible to confirm that the extra chromosome was a normal one, and suggested that the possibility of it being a fragment from another type of aberration could not be disregarded. I have referred to this caution in a recent conversation with Professor Lejeune, but he said: 'Oh, but I *knew*, yes, I *knew*, but who was going to believe me?'

In April of the same year two confirmatory reports were published. The first reported finding 48 chromosomes in a patient with both Down's and Klinefelter's syndrome. One of the supernumerary chromosomes was the extra X responsible for Klinefelter's syndrome, the other being the small chromosome which was consistent with Lejeune's findings in Down's syndrome. This paper actually placed the small extra chromosome with the pair now known as 22, although the authors did suggest that it could have been placed with pair 21, where in fact we know now that it did belong; these two smallest pairs are very similar.

The second report published the cytogenetic findings in four more cases of Down's syndrome, showing that one extra chromosome of the smallest size range was present. The authors of this paper noted that the supernumerary chromosome was clearly an autosome [1] and would probably have been of maternal origin.

By the following year, 1960, it had become clear exactly which chromosome was involved in the trisomy. Following on from the

1. A chromosome which is not a sex chromosome.

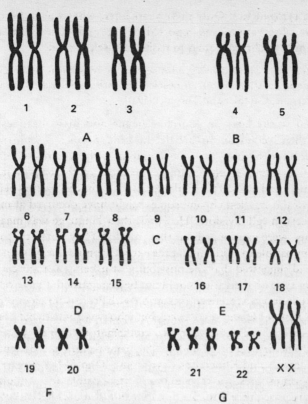

Figure 1. Karyotype of a standard trisomy 21 Down's syndrome (female) showing numbers and groups of chromosomes.

work of Tijo and Puck (1958) and Chu and Giles (1959), which was concerned with the description, grouping and numbering of individual pairs of chromosomes in the human genome,[1] Book and his associates studied three cases of Down's syndrome and reported that the extra chromosome was in fact number 21 (see Figure 1).

There was now no doubt that Down's syndrome, with all its characteristics, resulted from an extra chromosome on pair 21, but the story of Down's syndrome does not really begin with the discovery of its genetic foundations. The human story goes back many centuries.

1. The set of chromosomes found in the nucleus of the cell of a given species is referred to as the 'genome'.

CHAPTER 3

ATTITUDES AND ARTISTS

In ancient times

In the western world we proclaim Greece as the cradle of civilization and as the inventors of rule by the people, democracy. But which people, and just how civilized was Ancient Greece in modern terms? In fifth-century Athens there was a total population of 400,000, though its 'democracy' was maintained by half this population. The 200,000 slaves who made up the other half of the population certainly had no part in political life. Added to this it is necessary to consider the place of women in this fiercely male society. Women were little removed from the level of the slaves, with no public rights, even though a woman was required to be the daughter of a citizen in order to marry a citizen. The position of women in this society was summed up by Demosthenes: 'We have courtesans for our pleasure, concubines for our comfort and wives to give us legitimate children.' For the Athenian, his wife was merely the first of his servants.

Of course, in a democracy no one was compelled to take part in public life even when '*he*' had the right. He could elect to be a 'private person'. Naturally men were not encouraged to neglect their public duties, but it was accepted that one *could*, if one wished, be a 'private person'. The Greek word for a private person is 'idiot'. It became part of normal conversation in the late Hellenic period to suggest that a person who made a foolish statement was 'talking like an idiot', meaning of course one who is not aware of what is going on.

What little is known about the Greek attitude to the handicapped does them scant credit. The Athenians, like the Spartans, exposed handicapped children on the hillsides, either to die of starvation or to be devoured by wild animals. This deliberate neglect and abandonment was countenanced by the Laws of Lycurgus and was practised mainly from motives of eugenics (concern that developmental handicap should not be passed on), but also there seems to have been a fear of 'madmen' or those who might do things contrary to good Greek custom. There must have been some confusion between mental illness and mental handicap in that period. This confusion continued for a long time and is even today far from clear in the public mind.

The Greeks gave the word 'idiot' to the world and also its association with despised groups and stupidity. It is indeed strange that the word 'idiot' became an acceptable 'scientific' description for the severely mentally handicapped and was in frequent use until more than half-way into this century. Of course it also still remains with us but is now used more as a term of abuse.

However, not all societies in the ancient world regarded deformed or handicapped people in the same way. Survival of children with Down's syndrome would be rare, but it was most likely this rarity which, in contrast to the Ancient Greeks, made the Olmecs endow Down's syndrome with mystical, even supernatural qualities.

The Olmecs

The Olmecs were people who existed on about 7,000 square miles of alluvial plain around the Gulf of Mexico from about 1500 BC to AD 300. They have left sufficient artefacts to indicate that people bearing many kinds of abnormalities were held in great respect by them. So far, however, not a single human skeleton from this period has been found, and what is known about the people comes from their sculptures and figurines. It is possible that these Olmec sculptures have a religious significance and are more mythological than realistic, according to Reich (1979); but it still needs to be explained what the actual sources of these works of art might be. Even if they are idealizations and not 'portraits', there still had to be some human model as an inspirational source for the features in these sculptures, which one anthropologist has suggested are most unlikely to be part of the standard Olmec physical type.

Some scholars, dealing with the iconography of these works of art, have suggested that Olmec portable sculpture depicts either diseased individuals, or those whose body or facial features were markedly different from those which the Olmecs may have considered the norm. In contrast, Wicke, another anthropologist, has pointed out that the Olmec 'Colossal Heads' demonstrate that these people did have the technical skills necessary for realistic depictions. A Mexican anthropologist, Juan Comas, has concluded, after studying bone remains from other sites immediately outside the Olmec area, that the anthropomorphic representation in Olmec art is definitely not an expression of the normal Olmec type; they are, rather, 'exceptional cases which, *precisely because of their difference,* attracted the artist's attention.'

Children with Down's syndrome, with their distinctive appearance, would surely have been the subject of a great deal of curiosity among the Olmecs, who would have no explanation for their presence other than a supernatural one. More than one scholar, while linking the sculptured figures with symbolism and religion, agrees that an original source for the sculptures must have been 'abnormal' individuals. Certainly hunchbacks were regarded with some kind of reverence, judging by the number of reliefs, statues and figurines of all sizes which represent people with this deformity. A high incidence of spinal tuberculosis in the Olmec community has been suggested.

In the nearby Mayan region the rulers of Palenque suffered from the congenital defect of club foot. This is evident in a number of relief carvings. Greene-Robertson has concluded that the ruling class must have intermarried, since this is the only way that this abnormality could appear with such regularity in a lineage which lasted only about sixty years. The deformity was certainly not hidden by contemporary sculptors.

However, what is of particular interest are some representations of short, stocky figures tending to obesity, with round flat-cheeked faces, slanting puffy eyes, flat noses and open mouths with thick lips, heavy jaw line and very short, almost non-existent necks. The head shapes are generally flat at the back of the skull and tend to be on the small side. Some of these quartz figures also show hyperextensibility of the joints and have little or no genitalia, indicating sexual inactivity. These features make it difficult to conclude that the figures represent anything other than people with Down's syndrome. One such figure is of an adult person sucking his thumb, giving an impression of childlike behaviour. Covarrubias has stated that 'these beings seem to have concerned the people of this culture to the point that they must have worshipped them as supernatural beings – men perpetually children'. When the Spanish arrived in Mexico they commented that the Aztec rulers must have been surrounded by hunchbacks, dwarfs and children. Actually there is a more modern parallel which demonstrates that this kind of regard for handicapped people is not just fantasy. Only 100 years ago mentally handicapped people, in this case microcephalics (small-headed people), were maintained at a shrine in the Punjab. It was considered that they brought grace to the shrine and to its visitors. These mentally handicapped people were known, affectionately, as 'Shah Daula's rats'. In some parts of India this regard for handicapped people as having religious or mystical properties still maintains, and they are venerated at the shrines.

The American anthropologists Milton and Gonzalo, while maintaining that the Olmec tribes were careful observers of their gene pool, have proposed that the Olmec believed that these babies with Down's syndrome features resulted from the mating of a human with the Olmec's main totem, the jaguar; the offspring were therefore thought of as God-human hybrids by this civilization. Further weight may have been added to this belief if a high-placed and senior member of the tribe gave birth to a child with Down's syndrome; a situation which may well have arisen because of the increased age of the mother. Cave paintings at Oxotitlan lend credence to this assumption because they actually depict sexual relations between a jaguar and a human.

A healthy discussion rather than controversy continues to flourish around these figures; are they *really* representative of Down's syndrome, or is there some other explanation? I was certainly sceptical until I examined them in the company of an eminent professor of genetics while on a visit to the Museum of Anthropology in Mexico City. The search for more evidence goes on. It is unfortunate that no burial ground has been discovered from this period, as nothing is more convincing than skeletal remains, but the humid climate and the acidity of the soil have probably destroyed any such remains.

The Saxons

There is no doubt about a skull which was discovered in the 1950s during the excavation of a Saxon burial ground at Breedon-on-the-Hill in the County of Leicestershire in the United Kingdom. The skull has a shape and volume that falls well outside the range that could be expected in a normal Saxon population, but within the range of a modern European Down's syndrome population. Like the Olmec artefacts, the skull is brachycephalic (small) with a flattened occiput (back) and very thin vault; this would match a modern skull from a child with Down's syndrome, though there is no doubt that this child died and was buried in the ninth century. Other features of this Saxon skull are the short maxilla (upper jaw) but nearly normal mandible (lower jaw), which reflect typical characteristics of Down's syndrome, as do the small sinuses and dentition anomalies. Because disorganization of tooth and bone development occur with retarded brain development, it is difficult to give the age of death of this child, although it has been estimated that this skull is possibly that of a 9-year-old.

Breedon-on-the-Hill burial ground was probably associated with one of the larger monastic houses of the eighth or ninth century. It therefore becomes interesting to speculate that, with the spread of Christianity through Britain and the consequent greater attention to the sick and defective, the physically and mentally handicapped may have received help and protection at such places.

This was certainly true of the large monasteries in France where the mentally handicapped would gather to be fed and cared for. At this time and right through the Middle Ages there were large communities of people with hypothyroidism; tough, survivors, generally hard-working but quite severely mentally retarded. This condition was endemic in areas where there was a lack of iodine in the water. Also, as the condition is hereditary and these people were quite prolific 'breeders', there were large families of such handicapped people. Their social survival and maintenance would largely depend on the kindness of monastic communities. Some of the more able of these people were taken into the monastic community itself, to work as lay brothers. People who lived in the nearby villages would refer to these handicapped people who were living and working around the monastery as the Christians, or, as this was France, 'les Crétien', hence the origin of the name cretin. It is unfortunate that, like 'idiot', this name, so well meant at the time, has taken on a new meaning.

Among these would be the few surviving individuals with the condition now known as Down's syndrome, which has in the past been referred to as 'a softer kind of Cretinism'. It was probably a similar community at Breedon-on-the-Hill which had cared for the child with Down's syndrome who died at around the age of 9.

The Middle Ages, the Renaissance and later

In former ages the prospects of survival for any child, let alone the weak, were not very good. The late Thomas Weihs pointed out that in the Middle Ages, for instance, the average healthy woman would conceive many times but would carry to full term only perhaps about twelve children, of which maybe only two would survive. A number of children with Down's syndrome would be born, perhaps not to survive very long, but live birth incidence of Down's syndrome would not have undergone any dramatic changes since ancient times. Again, a few would survive beyond the first stage, at least into later childhood, and some of these have engaged the attention of painters; receiving special attention were those children born to noble families.

Artists from all periods have been impressed by the unusual, even the grotesque and the deformed are frequently recorded in a variety of media. The dwarf, for example, appears often in works of art. Representations of disease and physical deformity can be found in art form from ancient Greece to the Impressionists.

There is a painting of a *Madonna and Child* by Mantegna, painted when Mantegna was the court painter for the rich and powerful Gonzaga family in fifteenth-century Mantua. The child is undoubtedly a child with Down's syndrome.

Mantegna is an important figure in art history because, quite apart from his skills as a painter, he is considered to be a link between early mysticism and the later Renaissance. It is his keen eye for accuracy and his revolutionary approach to painting exactly what he perceived that gives more authenticity to this particular

Madonna and Child out of the many that he painted. This stands out as a painting of a child with Down's syndrome and of his mother. The child has the typical narrow openings to the eyes and the fold of skin on the eyelids. The nose is small with a depressed bridge and the tongue is protruding. The hands are broad and square with an inturned little finger. The space between the big and other toes is a compelling diagnostic feature.

In an article in one of the medical journals I have suggested that perhaps the model for the Madonna was a member of the Gonzaga family and that the child was in fact her own son. The model for this Madonna has a small goitre in her neck which suggests thyroid dysfunction, and the child also shows some signs of hypothyroidism as well as the more prominent features of Down's syndrome. Since the first suggestions, correspondence with a Roman art historian who had read the paper has thrown more light on this interesting painting. Dr Voci has pointed out that it is more likely that the Madonna is Nicolosa Bellini, the wife of Mantegna, and that the child with Down's syndrome belonged to them. It is known that Nicolosa had many children and lost most of them at a very early age. Four survived, but one who was sick (probably the child in the picture) also died, in spite of the efforts of Mantegna's patron Ludovico Gonzaga who tried to save the child's life by sending him to a famous doctor in Venice.

It has also been suggested, with some good evidence, that Ludovico and his wife Barbara di Brandenburgo themselves had a child with Down's syndrome, which might account in part for an apparent warm attachment between them and Mantegna. The speculation is that one of the ten children of Barbara di Brandenburgo, and the one likely to be the child with Down's syndrome, is depicted in the Mantegna painting of the *Presentation at the Temple*, where the mother of Jesus is modelled by Barbara. In this case the child presented may well be the same child who appears again in the famous painting *Gonzaga Family with Servants and Dwarf* in the Camera degli Sposi. This girl is then perhaps not a dwarf at all but the now grown daughter of the Gonzagas, the short stature being typical of Down's syndrome, as of course is the appearance. Dr Voci points out that the child is not dressed like a servant and is being looked upon with affection by others in the picture. From these paintings it may be assumed that the Mantegnas had a boy with Down's syndrome and the Gonzagas had a girl.

Survival of these children can be accounted for by the softer climate and the care which could be afforded by the richest family of the time. This makes a good story and of course historians could spend many happy hours disputing the relationships and identities of the subjects, but it is accepted by many physicians that the child held by the Madonna in Mantegna's painting is a child with Down's syndrome, some adding that there are also signs of cretinism, a not unusual phenomenon, as hypothyroidism can often occur along with Down's syndrome. The fact that such a painting could be produced says something about prevailing attitudes of the time. It is interesting to speculate on the reactions which might have erupted among the public today, even in our extremely secular age, if similar models were portrayed – what might be said if a great artist were to use a child with Down's syndrome as his model for Christ?

There are other examples of the influence which children with Down's syndrome have had on painters. I am indebted to Dr Patricia Sheehan of Dublin for pointing out the paintings of Filippo Lippi, a contemporary of Mantegna under the patronage of the de Medici. It is certain that Mantegna had visited Lippi in his studios in Florence and had been influenced by his work. There is one painting by Lippi of particular interest in the present context, because speculation about the angels surrounding a *Madonna della Humilità* painted by Lippi around 1437 draws attention to the unmistakable characteristics of Down's syndrome in their faces. It is doubtful that they were painted from models, for the rather chubby body features do not correspond with the hypotonic body of the typical infant with Down's syndrome; the faces, however, are almost archetypal. It is likely that Lippi was influenced by his early years, which were spent in an orphanage. It is here that he would have seen rejected babies and infants with Down's syndrome, and these children obviously made a lasting impression on the young Lippi. This painting now hangs in a gallery in Milan.

Artists are always keen observers, and it is a pity that they tend to leave very few written records of the intentions, feelings and reasons behind their choice of model. This absence of written record leaves room only for conjecture, as for example the proposal of Zellweger, an American paediatrician who suggested in the 1960s that an infant with Down's syndrome was represented in a painting by the Flemish artist Jacob Jordaens. This is again a painting on a religious theme, *The Adoration of the Shepherds*, painted by Jordaens in 1618; it depicts a woman holding a child with the characteristics of Down's syndrome. It has been suggested that the woman in this painting is Catherine van Noort, the artist's wife, and that the child is their daughter Elizabeth. The same child is used as a model in a number of paintings by Jordaens, so the features can be examined the same number of times. The results of these examinations lend more credence to the diagnosis of Down's syndrome in this child. A further notable example can be observed in one of Jordaens's secular paintings: *The Peasant and the Satyr*.

It is always necessary to exercise caution when looking at paintings from the distant past before making interpretations about the medical record of the subject without other supporting evidence. It is necessary to examine the style of the artist and to compare all his paintings. An illustration of this need for caution comes from a painting by Sir Joshua Reynolds. In 1774 Reynolds painted a portrait of *Lady Cockburn and her Children*. It has been proposed from time to time that one of the children, the one looking over his mother's shoulder, is a child with Down's syndrome. It has been pointed out in other sections of this book that some of the features of Down's syndrome, particularly heavy eyelids and a flattened nose bridge, are not unusual in all young children. What makes it extremely doubtful that this particular child painted by Reynolds was a child with Down's syndrome is the fact that it is now known that the same child later became an admiral in the British Navy, was knighted as Sir George Cockburn, and actually commanded the ship which in 1815 transported Napoleon to exile on St Helena. If this child had Down's syndrome it certainly beats any modern report of individuals with Down's syndrome passing their driving test! This, of course, is why it is necessary to be cautious in the interpretation of style.

Some artists were much more direct in their approach. There is a fascinating collection of paintings housed in the Castle Hradek near Nechanice in Czechoslovakia. The Spanish painter is unknown, but the paintings belong to the seventeenth century and were used as we might now use medical photography. They are fine portrait paintings executed with great artistic skill, but their purpose was to portray the physical characteristics of pathological features, just as today in any teaching hospital the photography is expected to be technically excellent even though the photographer would not expect his name to be known or his work to be reproduced in *Vogue*. Some of these portraits are quite grotesque. There is in this collection, however, a portrait of an adult man with an extremely jolly expression. The difference from the others is so striking that the gallery curator suggested to me that this might be a self-portrait of the artist. This, however, is not the case. It is quite obvious, and particularly in the context, that this is an illustration of an archetypal Down's syndrome adult. All the well-known facial features of Down's syndrome are illustrated in the picture as clearly as the exaggerated features of cretinism, gargoylism, hydrocephalus, hypertelorism, etc. are depicted in others. The seventeenth-century gentleman with Down's syndrome is well dressed in the fashion of the day; he is smiling widely, showing spaced teeth, and a flattened nose bridge and epicanthic folds to the eyes are well evident. He has a 'painted-on' (within the painting) moustache and beard, emphasizing of course the sparse hair growth in Down's syndrome, but also perhaps as an indication of his desire to be like the rest of the young men of his time. A very interesting feature of this painting is that the gentleman is wearing spectacles, yet it was not until well into this century that physicians began to make it clear that eyesight might be defective in the majority of people with Down's syndrome.

Apart from the Saxon skull from Breedon-on-the-Hill, which can be verified by anatomical examination as coming from a child with Down's syndrome, all this early material and 'evidence' comes from informed speculation, adding up evidence from sculptures, paintings and other artefacts. No one from these times has seen fit to distinguish the condition we now know as Down's syndrome in any of the writings which they have left, though the condition would certainly have existed and be familiar. Mental handicap as well as mental illness was well known, but only these two broad general categories would have any meaning. Even these categories were often confused until the fourteenth century, when it became necessary under the law to make a distinction between them (see page 38).

It was not until the nineteenth century that any attempts at differential diagnosis were made and began to appear in published form.

CHAPTER 4

EARLY MEDICAL AND SCIENTIFIC DESCRIPTIONS

The first written description of a person with Down's syndrome may have been made unwittingly by the French physician Jean-Etienne Esquirol, in a two-volume work on *Malades Mentales* published in Paris in 1838. Some doubt has been expressed as to whether Esquirol was in fact describing the particular condition we know now as Down's syndrome, since his language is rather fanciful and extravagant. Certainly his immoderate style was influenced by his belief that attempts at educating the mentally deficient were an unprofitable waste of time. He was quite adamant that 'Idiots are what they must remain for the rest of their lives.' Dr Esquirol could not, however, be described as an eccentric; he is regarded as one of the founders of modern psychiatry and was a very much respected figure in his day.

Nevertheless, his descriptions of the mentally handicapped are not only depressing but are presented without a glimmering of optimism about any kind of change for the better which might be expected. Esquirol recorded in the authoritative *Dictionnaire des sciences médicales:* 'Everything in them betrays a constitution that is imperfect, life forces misapplied. They are incurable . . .' He then goes on to present a graphic but depressing description of the mentally handicapped person. At that time, and under the prevailing living conditions within average mental institutions, his crude descriptions are undoubtedly accurate, but they remain very distressing to a modern-day reader. The complete lack of optimism is even worse. He goes on to describe these pitiable creatures inhabiting the asylums of France, who have reached 'the final stage of human degradation', in whom 'intellectual and moral faculties are devoid'. As to any form of treatment, the doctor is without hope:

The reader certainly anticipates that I have nothing to say about the treatment of a disease which is essentially incurable. To a certain extent one can improve the lot of imbeciles by accustoming them early on to some labour which can provide income for the poor imbecile or distraction for the rich one. But idiots only require attentive and intensive domestic care.

Of course times were different and the majority of ordinary people had to endure hardship and harsh living conditions. It was commonplace for mentally retarded individuals to be rejected by their families and simply abandoned, either to die or to live as best they could and in any way they might. It has been suggested that this current social treatment could have been the origin of the 'Wild Boy of Aveyron'. A certain degree of physical toughness was needed to survive under these conditions, and with their weaker constitution few children with Down's syndrome would have survived. The few who did survive beyond infancy would most likely have been placed in the kind of institutions from which Esquirol drew his conclusions. Any patient with Down's syndrome so existing might have fitted into his 'imbecile' category. In which case Esquirol's expectations of paid employment for these people were higher than they would be today!

Unfortunately, however, it is more likely that the impoverished environment, totally lacking in any form of mental stimulation, would have depressed the most determined person with Down's syndrome into the 'idiot' class – if for no reason other than that of a physical inability or 'intelligent' disinclination to carry out the kind of menial employment that would have been available to them. Some of the richer families *might* have kept a person with Down's syndrome at home, though 'shame' might have driven them to 'putting them away' into one of these institutions. The temperament of the person with Down's syndrome, their willingness to please and their potential for learning, given the right conditions, must have encouraged some of those who, while working in the field, did not see the prognosis of the mentally handicapped in the same terms as Esquirol.

One such was Jean-Marc Itard, a contemporary of Esquirol, and another was Édouard Séguin, a pupil of both of them. While there might have been recent doubts expressed that some of the descriptions by Esquirol of mentally handicapped people conformed to Down's syndrome, there can be no doubt about the subject of Séguin's description, written in 1846.

Édouard Séguin was the last pupil of Itard, the physician well known for his attempts to educate the 'Wild Boy of Aveyron'. Though disappointed with the results of his efforts, Itard remained a firm believer in the treatment of mental disability through educational methods, and he passed on his enthusiasm to his pupil. Getting on in years and too sick to attend to the last patient presented to him, Itard offered the care of this patient to a more youthful colleague, with the words, 'If I were younger, I would undertake his care; but send me someone suitable and I will direct his efforts.' Séguin's name was suggested, to which Itard replied, 'If Séguin will accept, I will answer for the result.'

The 25-year-old Séguin, later to be called the 'Apostle of the Idiots', took up the challenge.

His later description of this first patient is now generally accepted to be that of Down's syndrome:

... milky white, rosy, and peeling skin; with its shortcomings of all the integuments which give an unfinished aspect to the truncated fingers and nose; with its cracked lips and tongue, with its red ectopic conjuctiva, coming out to supply the curtained skin at the margin of the lids.

Séguin's progress after a year and a half's work with this patient gave him the encouragement he needed to carry on his work with the mentally handicapped with renewed confidence. Even Dr Esquirol, in an ungrudging gesture, put his name to an affidavit testifying to Séguin's success. Esquirol was:

... pleased to affirm that M. Édouard Séguin, born at Clamecy, has begun, with the greatest success, the education of a child almost mute and apparently an idiot – by reason of the limited development of his intellectual and moral faculties. In eighteen months, M. Séguin has taught his pupil to make use of his senses, to remember, to compare, to speak, to write, to count, etc. This training was conducted by M. Séguin following the method of the late Dr Itard, from whom he received his inspiration.

Édouard Séguin's career started by training one mentally handicapped child, a child who was more than probably a child with

Down's syndrome. It ended by influencing thousands upon thousands of handicapped children throughout Europe and the United States of America.

Later theories and classifications

Few, if any, specific descriptions appeared in the literature during the next twenty years. Mental handicap was at this time regarded as one single condition and was classified according to the degree of its severity. Attempts at differential diagnosis were not made in any systematic way until the time when Langdon Down published his famous paper in 1866. Before this paper was published, but in the same year, there appeared a description – which could refer only to Down's syndrome – in a London publication under the title of 'A manual for classification, training and education of the feeble-minded imbecile and idiotic'. The description was of a girl with '. . . a small round head, Chinese-looking eyes, projecting lower lip and large tongue, who knew only a few words but could sing'.

It is important to remember that while the majority of physicians were describing the characteristics of mentally handicapped people and debating treatment, others in the early nineteenth century were discussing the genesis of mental deficiency itself. The weight of scholarly opinion in this respect and at this time was in favour of a theory of degeneracy, intractable mental deficiency being caused by some kind of atavistic regression, a kind of throw-back to a more primitive form of existence. It took courage to dispute these prevailing theories upheld by the most influential scholars of the time; this makes all the more admirable the work of people like Itard and Séguin who had carefully examined conventional wisdom and had seen its shortcomings.

A firm upholder of the degeneracy theory was Chambers, who made sweeping generalizations about the nature of mental deficiency in his book *The Vestiges of the Natural History of Creation*, published in 1844. He also made an attempt at classification. It was in this book that possibly the first-ever reference to Down's syndrome as 'mongolian' was made. This was twenty-two years before Langdon Down was to make the same analogy. Chambers wrote with conviction but quite mistakenly: 'It is found that parents too nearly related tend to produce offspring of the Mongolian type.' He then thought it worth informing his readers that this means '. . . persons who in maturity still are a kind of children'. Chambers continued to elaborate the degeneracy theory: 'In the Caucasian or Indo-European family alone has the primitive organization been improved upon. The Mongolian, Malay, American and Negro, comprehending perhaps five-sixths of mankind, are degenerate.'

Of course this was the time of British supremacy, the height of Empire! At that time it would have been quite natural arrogantly to assume that the further away from London they were, the more primitive a population must be. At such a time the degeneracy theory would have had popular appeal. It is interesting to note that the same condition had been observed at about the same time in Mongolia and had been described as 'the European disease'!

This then was the political, social and scientific climate against which John Langdon Down proposed a classification of different manifestations of mental handicap in his celebrated paper, 'Observations on an ethnic classification of idiots', which he published in the *London Hospital Reports* in 1866. The paper was based on his observations at the Earlsfield Hospital. Langdon Down described five classes of patients: Caucasian, Ethiopian, Malay, American and Mongolian, but he paid particular attention to the 'Mongolian' class. He meticulously described the characteristics of this type of patient; the face, hair, skin and mental condition. Echoing the scientific reasoning of his day, he accepted that these features were due to atavistic degeneration, but he attempted to bring some further rationalization and reasoning into the classification. Far from causing a sensation, Langdon Down's paper was just accepted and then generally ignored. He had said nothing startlingly new, and his analysis was a little too indulgent for popular taste.

Taken out of context of its time, Langdon Down's explanation would certainly seem to have racist overtones. It is perhaps due to this and the fact that Langdon Down is always and exclusively associated with the now rejected term 'mongol' that he has had a good deal of unfavourable criticism in modern times. Much of this criticism is unfair, because a different picture emerges if his paper is read alongside the imperialistic writings of Chambers and others in the nineteenth century. Langdon Down goes on to suggest that 'these human examples of racial retrogression' were proof that racial divisions were not fixed and unsurmountable, but could easily be broken down by disease. He completes his paper with the words:

> These examples of the results of degeneracy among mankind appear to me to furnish some argument in favour of the unity of the species.

Langdon Down was offering a much more compassionate way of looking at the currently accepted theory. He later used this same argument when declaring his opposition to Negro slavery in the Southern States of America. Langdon Down had been influenced early in his student days by the work of Blumenbach, a celebrated social anthropologist of the time who was interested in ethnographical classification. This early influence must have had a profound effect on Langdon Down's own thinking and on his subsequent theories concerning the condition which was eventually to take his name.

Dr Langdon Down was a highly respected physician with an enviable professional reputation. Many of his friends and colleagues were dismayed when they learned that he intended to devote his career to the 'idiots', 'imbeciles' and 'feeble-minded' who inhabited the asylums and who were given at that time very low priority by the medical profession. Indeed, there were some practitioners who believed that such conditions were no business of theirs. How could mental deficiency belong in the province of doctors? After all, knowledge about them was rudimentary, treatment was almost non-existent and conditions in asylums were anything but good. Nonetheless, Langdon Down committed himself exclusively to working with these rejects of that society. A recent article in the *Practitioner* has gone some way towards restoring Langdon Down's reputation, describing him as 'a most kind and compassionate man'.

Langdon Down's reformist views are demonstrated in one of his later discursive publications, not concerned with the mentally deficient, where he looks forward to a future when women would not be just 'mothers of men', but 'also companions and helpers of men'.

In this work he defended the higher education of women, rejecting the popular notion of the time that pursuing the demands of higher education would make women more likely to produce feeble-minded children. Although Langdon Down's ideas could hardly be considered as shockingly liberal by today's standards, in the late nineteenth century such views would have been considered almost immoral.

After Dr John Langdon Down

Even though, as we are now aware, Langdon Down's reasoning about causes was incorrect, the scientific writers who followed him all gave him the credit for having isolated a new and quite distinct clinical entity. A 'new' condition now needed to be identified by a new name. Apart from those names popularly applied to the condition as a result of the association which had been made by Langdon Down and those before him, such as mongol, mongolism, mongolian, mongolian idiocy, mongolian imbecile, mongolian deformity, other names began to be used which, perhaps more appropriately, connected the name of Langdon Down with the condition. An interesting link was made initially with the man first known to have described such a patient; the condition was at that time sometimes referred to as the Séguin-Down syndrome.

As so often happens in the history of scientific discovery, not long after its first disclosure as a separate entity Down's syndrome was 'discovered' again. Ten years later (it must be acknowledged that exchange of scientific information was not so rapid in those days) two others, Fraser and Mitchell, claimed in a paper to be the first to have described the condition. Obviously they had not read the 1866 *London Hospital Reports*.

The Fraser and Mitchell paper is interesting for two reasons. First, they had independently come to the same conclusion as Langdon Down, i.e. that the problem was somehow connected with 'racial regression'. They described the condition as 'Kalmuck Idiocy'. The Kalmucks, physically small as a race, were members of a confederacy of Buddhist Mongol tribes originating in Sungaria, most of them returning there early in the nineteenth century after making their homes on the lower Volga for about two centuries.

Fraser and Mitchell also illustrate in their paper the foot, showing the wide space between the big and other toes. This characteristic of the foot is naturally a less obvious but possibly one of the most distinctive and important diagnostic features of Down's syndrome. While very few 'normal' people have this space between the toes, more than 90 per cent of those with Down's syndrome carry the feature. The second reason for interest in Fraser and Mitchell's paper is that it contains the first published drawing, photograph or etching of a person with Down's syndrome. The illustration is of a well-dressed, well-groomed young man and is a much more agreeable and acceptable representation than some 'institutionalized' illustrations which appear in medical text books of the 1930s.

The 'degeneracy' or 'regression' theory, erroneous as it so obviously was, has probably had more influence on beliefs and attitudes towards people with Down's syndrome than any other hypothesis. The conviction that the condition was linked with a more 'primitive' race was strongly held, and this remained as an acceptable explanation far longer than did less outrageously false theories. More than half a century after Langdon Down had offered his theories of 'mongolism', an even more offensive theory was proposed and with far less justification. Crookshank, writing in 1924, suggested that the earlier writers had not gone far enough back in terms of regression. The 'mongol' was, he proclaimed, sub-human and could be traced beyond a Mongolian ancestry to the anthropoid animal kingdom; he implicated the *orangutan*. An interesting and lingering legacy of this highly objectionable theory is still present in the medical description given to the single crease across the palms of people with Down's syndrome. This feature is known as the 'simian' crease. 'Simian' literally means pertaining to the apes or monkeys. However, it is difficult to accommodate to this theory the fact that a fair percentage of the 'normal' population also carry this distinctive crease!

Links with other conditions

Of course the fact that Down's syndrome had first been linked with the much more common condition of cretinism continued to influence medical descriptions. Séguin had suggested the name 'furfuraceous cretin' for the patient he had described. Presumably he was trying to imply a 'softer' kind of cretinism. Something of the agreeable personality of people with Down's syndrome was already beginning to be recorded in descriptions. It might be said that observations of this nature are much more significant in terms of human values than those of appearance, which can frequently be superficial.

Some time ago the late Dr Thomas Weihs, a physician, Austrian by birth, who worked for many years with the mentally handicapped, spoke of this difference in a moving way when he made reference to children with Down's syndrome in delivering a public lecture on 'Children in Need of Special Care' at Leeds University in 1977. He spoke of a period of increase in numbers of children with Down's syndrome and contrasted this with a decline in cretinism:

As you see, about the time when the mongol child appeared, the Cretin disappeared because we have found that it is a thyroid disfunction caused by a deficiency in iodine; and by adding iodine to the salt in the mountain countries where there was deficiency of iodine the endemic Cretinism had disappeared. Could it not be that mankind needed the Cretin as a kind of forerunner to lead us towards our more intellectual orientation? To lead us to learn to plan, to consider cause and effect, to make possible what we call progress . . .

It is also fitting that we do not lose sight of moral values as we pursue scientific explanations. There were, however, good scientific reasons for maintaining the connection with cretinism and these were not finally dispelled until well into the 1950s; but that is a story which belongs in another chapter.

Temperament and disposition are subjects which have influenced descriptions since Down's syndrome began to be reported. They continue to form part of any discussion about Down's syndrome today, regardless of the specific aspect of Down's syndrome under consideration. Sutherland voiced the personality difference between Down's syndrome and cretinism as early as 1900. Eloquently summarizing his impressions of the two conditions, he wrote:

The smiling face of the Mongolian imbecile suggests the possession of some secret source of joy, while the somewhat sad countenance of the cretin suggests the cherishing of a secret sorrow.

It is, however, now well established that these are two quite distinctive and unrelated afflictions, though it is of course possible for a child to be born with Down's syndrome and *also* with cretinism. Down's syndrome of itself does not preclude being born with additional disabling conditions. Fortunately, however, the majority of children born with Down's syndrome do not have the problem of a second syndrome.

After Langdon Down's paper, the syndrome he had described became the subject of an increasing number of investigations, and while the majority of writers referred to the subjects of their studies as 'mongols' (or some variation of 'mongol'), other names were suggested from time to time, always indicating some uneasiness with the 'racial' description even early in the century. Among those suggested were some highly complicated and now fairly meaningless names – acromicria, generalized foetal displasia, peristatic amentia, for example – but the name 'mongol' had become firmly established.

Trisomy 21 had been gaining some favour since Lejeune's discovery and particularly in France, but Down's syndrome seems to be the name which is almost universally accepted and which is recognized by the majority of people. It should be noted that there is a move, particularly in the United States but coming officially from the World Health Organization, to drop the apostrophe 's', though this seems to be sheer pedantry, apart from being difficult to distinguish in spoken English.

CHAPTER 5

EARLY SEARCH FOR A CAUSE

In the early days of medicine, physicians were as concerned with the aetiology (cause) of a disease as they are today. Explanations suggesting causes of mental handicap have always been abundant, varied and sometimes contradictory. Some of the explanations of causes go back many centuries and owe their existence more to religion and philosophy than they do to medicine. At the time, of course, theology and medicine were a great deal closer than they are today.

The attitude of the Greeks towards handicapped people has been described in an earlier chapter. The extreme indifference the Greeks showed towards handicapped people, putting recognizably handicapped babies to death in barbaric ways and showing no humanity to those who did live into adulthood, is partly explained by the belief held in the fourth and third centuries BC that such creatures were not human but were 'monsters' belonging to another species. It was Aristotle who counselled differently, explaining that they were human and belonged to the *natural* order. However, Aristotle offered no suggestion of cause or explanation for their existence.

Possibly the earliest explanation put forward to account for the existence of mental handicap was the Augustinian notion that feeble-mindedness was associated with the fall of Adam. It is perhaps worth spending a few moments examining St Augustine's explanation because it has often been open to misinterpretation. These interpretations have led to the belief that St Augustine maintained that mental handicap comes about as a result of sins, particularly those of the parents. That parents are in some way culpable is a superstition which has tended not to diminish or disappear with time, as many other beliefs which originated in superstitions have done. This undefinable sense of guilt which seems to be seeking self-punishment is behind a good deal of quite unnecessary distress felt by parents. The idea that parents are being punished for sins previously committed was obviously already a well-established assumption in the fifth century because St Augustine was at pains to dispel the notion.

While the question of causes of misfortune, disease and corruption is frequently raised in the works of St Augustine, he draws particular attention to handicapped children in a letter to Jerome, a priest living in Jerusalem in the year 415. Attempting to answer the eternal question, 'Why does God permit . . .?' St Augustine writes that it has sometimes been said that 'in this way the sins of parents are either made known or punished', but he goes on to challenge this notion, pointing out that when God made man in His own image, everything was in a state of perfection, but as a result of man's disobedience in the Garden of Eden, not only sin but all other torments, sorrows and tribulations came into the world. God had not created evil; evil resulted from the fall of Adam. The significant sin was *original* sin and not the individual wrong-doings of those who followed Adam. A particularly poignant passage in St Augustine's letter makes reference to his own difficulties in coming to terms with the problem: 'But, when I come to the question of the sufferings of infants, believe me I am beset with great trouble, and I find no ready answer.' He goes on to try to find a 'just cause' for the suffering of children and says, 'Certainly there must be proof that they suffer all this justly, but without any evil cause on their part. Therefore a just cause must be assigned to these great sufferings which befall little children.'

St Augustine reasons that the same principles cannot be applied to children as to adults. He points out that Job's goodness was being tested and Herod's sins were being punished, but virtue cannot be being tested in young children. St Augustine cannot find an answer, but he is sure that neither they nor their parents are being punished.

St Augustine's writings come close to responding to those hidden fears, worries and concerns which are timeless. Even today some communities exist where a barely concealed expression is given that a mentally handicapped child results from 'the sins of the fathers'.

Explanations for the causes of mental handicap introduced by St Augustine were reflected in the mid-sixteenth-century work of Paracelsus entitled *The Begetting of Fools*. Paracelsus was at pains to describe the mature deficiency and its relationship to the body and the soul, and, like St Augustine before him, had regard to the place of people so afflicted in the teachings and philosophy of the Church. Paracelsus was particularly anxious to describe God's protection for the mentally handicapped, their influence for the good of others and their eventual redemption.

Not all were so compassionate as St Augustine or the later Paracelsus. Mental deficiency continued to be associated with evil spirits and sin. There was a strong belief that the mentally handicapped were possessed by the devil or somehow connected with witchcraft and consequently they were frequently burnt at the stake. There was no need to search for a cause, it was perfectly clear that the devil was involved. There was no doubt in the mind and teaching of Martin Luther, who firmly believed that mentally handicapped children came about as punishment for the sins of individual parents, and he was not impressed by the arguments of St Augustine and his followers that it was *original* sin which caused all our trials and tribulations. Luther was quite adamant that mentally handicapped children were born to those who did not love God or fear Him enough; or because their parents had been promiscuous and had given birth to illegitimate children, or were adulterers or indulged in thinking bad thoughts.

The mother was thought to be especially to blame. It was even fairly common belief at this time that a mentally handicapped child could have resulted from sexual intercourse with the devil. It is instructive to compare this belief with the Olmecs' belief around 3,000 years earlier that such children resulted from intercourse with their totem, the jaguar; though the attitude of the Olmecs took the opposite viewpoint and they celebrated the infant as a sacred person. However, the theme, or underlying belief, was essentially the same. But in Europe, such a birth with its surrounding superstitions gave good grounds for condemning the mother as a witch. What could be expected from such an evil liaison? Luther preached that the devil then substituted himself in place of a human child and therefore the child could not have a soul. Luther wrote:

'The devil sits in such changelings where the soul should have been.' He suggested that they should be put to death. This was a return to the 'monstrous' belief of the ancient Greeks. The Austrian psychologist, Jung, was later to take up this theme, describing such connections as belonging to 'the great racial unconscious', explaining why remote peoples in different times held similar kinds of fantasies and beliefs.

The Middle Ages, then, was marked by cruelty to the handicapped and to their families. Paradoxically, however, there was also a great deal of tenderness evident, such as was shown to the babies with Down's syndrome by the Gonzagas of Mantua and by those monastic communities who gave such love and care and protection to handicapped people. These, however, were either the high-placed or the fortunate few. The majority of handicapped people would have had a very difficult time in the Middle Ages.

The influential and wealthy were more able to protect handicapped members of their families. They were able to secure the best treatments, such as were available and even ineffective though they might be. At any event it is unlikely that the cause of handicap would be diagnosed as diabolical possession for people in high and influential positions. The rich did have another problem, however; they possessed land. If the handicapped person was to be in a position to inherit, then some protection of the inheritance was needed. It was not so much the cause of the condition which created the problem, it was more the nature of the condition itself. Confusion continuously existed between those who were intractably handicapped and those who had temporary lapses of social competence and mental ability. A distinction needed to be made between mental handicap and mental illness. Clarification became necessary, and finally was incorporated into one of the earliest laws of the land.

In the reign of Edward II, the prerogatives of the King were set out in the Statutes (*De praerogativa regis*, 1325) defining the difference between mental handicap and mental illness. It was relatively easy to distinguish the idiots, they were 'natural fools' (*fatuorum naturalium*), and the King's prerogative was set out to protect their lands.

Defining the mentally ill was more problematic; sometimes they were well and perfectly normal but sometimes they were incapable of taking care of themselves. In other words and in the words of the early English translation of the Latin text, they 'wax and wain as doth the moon wax and wain'. The analogy with the moon gave them the name 'lunatics'. The law now was to 'provide for the safe keeping of the lands of the lunatics so that the lands might be restored to them when they came of right mind'. From this time until the nineteenth century there was to be no confusion between the mentally handicapped and the mentally ill.

Among ordinary people idiots fared best in the villages. No one asked the cause; the 'village idiot' was accepted and cared for by the community. The majority of the population were uneducated, so differences in ability would be recognized only in terms of social competence. Also there would be few idiots among the poor. Infant mortality was high and it would be unusual for a weak child, such as one with Down's syndrome, to survive. The most common and likely cause of 'idiocy' in these handicapped survivors in the villages would be cretinism. For the rich, who would have been privately tutored, intelligence tests were eventually devised in order to determine that their level of ability placed them in the category of 'incompetents'. The same test was applied to both the mentally handicapped and the mentally ill. These tests, devised in the sixteenth century, must have been the first intelligence tests ever constructed. They were very simple and unsophisticated tests. Fitzherbert's test, produced in 1534, required the subject to know his age, the names of his parents and also to be able to count out twenty pence. Swinburne revised the test in 1591, including the ability to measure a yard of cloth and to name the days of the week.

In Elizabethan times, a period of social change, many of the poorer handicapped people along with others were beginning to find life in the villages less supportive. The old feudal system had started to decline, and the 'handicapped' began a migration towards the towns and cities. So the *mentally* handicapped were now beginning to be classed with these drifters: the beggars, cripples, paupers, petty criminals. The workhouse was eventually introduced as a means of coping with this motley crowd. Institutionalization of the mentally handicapped had begun.

The workhouse was the forerunner of the mental institution, or lunatic asylum. Many of the same categories of people who were inhabiting the workhouses were to find their way into the lunatic asylums; diagnosis of mental deficiency was fairly primitive. It is ironic that a decline in neighbourly tolerance and charitable concern for the mentally handicapped should herald a rise in interest in treatment of the handicapped and a renewed interest in searching for causes.

The idea of degeneration, which was eventually to lead to the description of Down's syndrome as mongolism, began to creep into theories of causes of mental handicap as early as the seventeenth century when Willis, an English doctor, proposed that something must have gone wrong in the parents' reproductive system. He further proposed that this cause was associated with immoral behaviour, or if there had been no immoral behaviour then by too much studying; either indulgence causing a weakening of the mind. The likely result would be weak-minded or mentally deficient children. With varying degrees of 'scientific' sophistication, this same notion persisted through the eighteenth and nineteenth centuries.

CHAPTER 6

LATER SEARCH FOR A CAUSE

Seeking for a cause rather than just an explanation of mental handicap became the preoccupation of a new 'scientific' approach which began in the nineteenth century. The idea of parental sin, however, far from being removed as a causal factor, became even more embedded as a result of actual and defined sins being assumed into 'scientific' reasoning. Mental deficiency was seen as a consequence of social evils, and 'sin' figured largely in the reasoning. Early in the nineteenth century, one writer referred to a large class of people who ignored health and reason and 'consequently sin in various ways'. Such sins, he reasoned, would have an effect on the state of the child, causing such a child to be constitutionally feeble-minded. Thus, biological factors were now inextricably linked with former religious and moral factors.

It was against this kind of background that the new eugenics movement was to arise, with its disturbing reasoning, based loosely on social Darwinism. The movement, with its startling 'revelations', set back the study of human genetics so far that we have not yet fully recovered from it to this day. The study of genetics is tainted by some of the preposterous deductions which were made at that time and which eventually were to find terrifying practical application in the holocaust perpetrated in Nazi Germany. It is not without significance that the oldest and most prestigious scientific journal concerned with human genetics changed its name after the Second World War from the *Annals of Eugenics* to the *Journal of Human Genetics*.

The means of studying large groups of mentally handicapped people had come about as a result of bringing them together in lunatic asylums. Now irrational fears began to be spread, through the publication of lectures and so-called scientific studies of the causes of mental deficiency. One important and influential publication just after the turn of the century sums up the currently accepted belief as to the main causes, pointing out frequently the social and economic burden of the mentally handicapped. The report states that

... the feeble-minded are a parasitic, predatory class ... They cause unutterable sorrow at home and are a menace and danger to the community. Feeble-minded women are invariably immoral and if at large become carriers of venereal disease or give birth to children who are as defective as themselves. The feeble-minded woman who marries is twice as prolific as the normal woman.

Of course there was no supportive evidence for these statements. They were based on the flimsiest kind of scientific reasoning which would be laughable to a present-day schoolchild taking GCSE science subjects. A typical example is how they deduced that pauperism must be hereditary, because 'there are families who have been paupers for many generations'.

A depressing and totally false belief springing from this time, which must have influenced later attitudes to the handicapped, maintained that all mentally handicapped people were potential criminals only waiting for the opportunity to express their innate criminal tendencies.

That this terrifying and intolerant attitude took root in public credibility can be seen from a report by Brinkworth. Residents of a village in north-east England protested vigorously at a proposal for a group home for adults with Down's syndrome, and told a local planning committee that 'all grades of mongols have committed murder and acts of violence'. They pointed out that such a house and its grounds would have to be made extremely secure so that their own children would be safe. This was in 1984!

Fortunately, all investigators in the nineteenth and early twentieth centuries were not carried away by the outrageous theories of a few fanatics who did untold damage to the rational study of the causes of mental handicap. Sound reasoning and objective research went on, even if the background against which it was conducted was often, by today's standards, unreasonable. Attempts were beginning to be made to differentiate different types and forms of mental handicap and to trace causes and pathological differences.

Once the 'mongolian' type of mental handicap had been isolated, physicians of the day were soon to spend a great deal of time and effort in the search for a cause of this type of disability, particularly as there seemed at the time to be a quite dramatic increase in numbers of these newly described 'mongols'. Consequently, many theories were proposed and, where possible, investigated.

Down's syndrome is associated with the extra chromosome on pair 21. This discovery, made in 1959 by Lejeune and his colleagues, has been described in an earlier chapter. However, even though this is now familiar and has been acknowledged for some thirty years, it is still by no means clear which biological or physical process causes non-disjunction of those chromosomes to come about. The theories behind the many earlier investigations, prior to the 1959 discovery, are interesting in themselves and for the influence they had on the development of attitudes as well as fostering further study and debate.

It has been stated previously that a good deal of confusion existed between the conditions of Down's syndrome and cretinism. This was not attributable to appearance alone, although undoubtedly the appearance of cretinism, like Down's syndrome, is very obvious. This appearance played a large part in determining attitudes to these people. Large communities of cretins existed in Switzerland, where the mountain water was deficient in iodine (a prime cause of cretinism), and travellers in that part of the world often remarked on their presence, though rarely with tolerance or sympathy. They would focus their attention on the 'ugliness' of these people and on their peculiar behaviour, and would frequently deduce, as was the fashion, that immorality was bound to follow, these creatures being classed as less than human. Yet to those who lived among them, the cretins were regarded as being without sin and as a blessing from God. Ryan and Thomas, writing of these people today, have stated that a family who did not have a cretin was somehow regarded as being out of favour with heaven. Brian Kirman has also reported that they were given high status in the community and were frequently described as 'Les enfants du bon Dieu'.

Classification

By the late nineteenth century mental handicap had been divided into three types, according to supposed causes, namely 'accidental', 'congenital' and 'developmental'. 'Accidental' is easily accounted for by brain damage caused by accident or disease (e.g. post-encephalitis, meningitis) and occurring after birth. Down's syndrome is obviously not in this category because it occurs at the moment of conception. However, when the descriptions of 'congenital' and 'developmental' types were studied, it could be seen even then that the difference was merely one of degree and not of kind. If factors which caused 'congenital idiocy' occurred after the sixth or seventh month of embryonic development, they rightly reasoned that 'developmental idiocy' would result. Hence, the division was somewhat arbitrary. It was suggested in a clinical lecture by Shuttleworth in 1886 that the problem could be resolved by using just two categories, 'congenital' and 'non-congenital'. Even so, this neither satisfied nor explained the profound distinction that actually exists between Down's syndrome (a congenital problem) and cretinism (a developmental problem). In fact, the confusion between these two disorders is demonstrated by the fact that tabulated descriptions were still being published in the *Lancet* and the *British Medical Journal*, distinguishing 'mongols' and 'cretins', well after the turn of the century. A supposed relationship was still worthy of comment in the 1920s, and indeed, thyroid dysfunction, which is at the basis of cretinism, was discussed in connection with Down's syndrome in the 1960s.

It was fairly widely accepted by the end of the nineteenth century that whatever the causal factors of Down's syndrome might be, they must have made their impression on the foetus, for the simple reason that, unlike cretinism, Down's syndrome was clearly present at birth.

Many physicians of this later nineteenth-century era believed that the unusual appearance of a child with Down's syndrome was caused by slower than normal development before birth, forty weeks seeming just not long enough for the development to become complete. This was not an unreasonable assumption to make; after all, development was manifestly slow after birth. Shuttleworth attempted to express this particular and observable pathological feature by coining the description of the child with Down's syndrome as 'the unfinished child'. Even in our own time, Weihs has said of the child with Down's syndrome that he is 'open to the scrutiny of others as is no other child, being *born insufficiently clothed of body*'.

In fact this whole concept may not be in as great a conflict with Down's original regression theory as it at first appears, especially when taking into account the popular interest which was being taken in Darwin's theories which were circulating at that time. Darwin had suggested that the embryo reflects the evolution of the species during its development in the uterus. In this respect it is interesting to contemplate the appearance of any three- to four-month embryonic development; all of us have something of the image of the child with Down's syndrome at this stage of development. It is this fact which gave rise to the short-lived theory that Down's syndrome arose from a neoteny; that is, a kind of incomplete development which happens sometimes among lower forms of life, the tadpole which grows up as a tadpole without becoming a frog, or the chrysalis which does not complete its development to the butterfly stage.

Disease

The first mention of any causal relationship between disease and Down's syndrome was made in Langdon Down's original paper, where he noted:

> The tendency is to the tuberculosis, which I believe to be the hereditary origin of the degeneration.

The idea of familial tuberculosis being the cause of Down's syndrome became a popular early theory. Shuttleworth, whose work has previously been mentioned, was a well-known figure in the field of Down's syndrome. He pointed out that one third of his patients with Down's syndrome had a family history of tuberculosis. Shuttleworth referred to pre-1866 casebooks at Earlswood Asylum which mentioned a 'strumerous' (i.e. tubercular) type of cretin. He also reported that 60 per cent of families who had a child with Down's syndrome also had a history of tuberculosis. Other investigators of the time also mention the 'preponderating influence of tuberculosis' in parents or grandparents of children with Down's syndrome. There is also frequent mention of a tuberculosis-like ill health in the mothers of these children.

Sutherland, however, writing in 1900, dismissed tuberculosis as a possible cause. He announced that, 'Amongst such possible diseases, tuberculosis has been suggested, but a parental history of that affliction does not stand out predominantly amongst my cases.' Later, even Shuttleworth reconsidered his earlier confidence in the influence of tuberculosis as a factor in the aetiology of Down's syndrome, noting that tuberculosis was 'common in all cases of imbecility'. In fact in the late nineteenth century tuberculosis was common in the whole population, handicapped or not.

Emotional Stress

The effect of emotional stress in the mother preceding a Down's syndrome birth was considered to be of some importance by Langdon Down. This particular issue is of interest because it is a factor which has also been implicated in more recent studies.

In 1961 Stott reported that he had found a highly significant excess of 'emotional shock' (i.e. those shocks which are more related to fear, grief or distress and not to minor accidents or falls) to have occurred during the first trimester of pregnancy in mothers of children with Down's syndrome as compared with other mothers. The data from which these findings are extracted were obtained from questionnaires completed only by members of MENCAP (Society for Mentally Handicapped Children), and because of this restriction the results have been widely criticized.

Many of the critics maintained that little credence could be given to histories of emotional stress which were obtained in retrospect, since mothers of handicapped children are more likely to search backwards for a possible cause for their child's condition. It was also pointed out that histories of maternal stress should always be discounted because they cannot be properly evaluated. The most important criticism of this research, however, is that there is no differentiation between the reported stress in mothers as to whether it was pre-conceptual or post-conceptual. Clearly, however traumatic the stress, if it had occurred post-conceptually it could not in any way have influenced a Down's birth. Even allowing for these quite reasonable criticisms of the research method and the questionable validity of the research results, the phenomenon of emotional stress as a factor in 'abnormal' births cannot be entirely ruled out, since it is known that emotional stress in women can disturb the balance of hormones.

A further and more searching study was later carried out in Edinburgh by two scientists whose findings confirmed those of Stott. They reported that the emotional stress factors were particularly marked in mothers aged 40 and over. However, there was a difference; these new findings placed the significant period of stress as *pre-conceptual* in origin.

Such is the nature of scientific inquiry, however, that the results of another investigation carried out by Professor Campbell Murdoch in New Zealand and reported in 1985 contradicted these findings. Murdoch presented convincing evidence that equal hormonal disturbances could be found both in mothers of children with Down's syndrome and mothers of non-handicapped children; the disturbances were evident before and *after* the birth of their children. Campbell Murdoch concluded that having a baby and attending to the demands of a new baby can be emotionally stressful periods for anyone! The prolonged effect of emotional strain on mothers of children with Down's syndrome has yet to be investigated.

Some 'discreditable' or 'unsavoury' causes suggested

Just before the turn of the century some other, rather less socially acceptable, theories were debated as possible relevant factors in the aetiology of Down's syndrome. Hereditary syphilis was still held by some to have a degree of responsibility for Down's syndrome, even though the hypothesis was already being rejected in 1886.

In the last of three lectures delivered to the Medical Society of London in 1886 and published the same year in the *British Medical Journal*, Professor Jonathan Hutchinson, a surgeon and authority on venereal diseases, spoke about the supposed 'connection' between mental deficiency and inherited syphilis but stated quite emphatically that syphilis could not be connected to Down's syndrome. Langdon Down had in fact referred some of his patients to Professor Hutchinson for his advice and opinion.

Some confusion arose in diagnosis and consequent theories of causes because of certain similarities in secondary afflictions which were associated with syphilis. Children with Down's syndrome could and generally did have eye problems, dentition problems and hearing problems. Perhaps there were children with Down's syndrome who by chance also had inherited syphilis and this would even further confuse the issue; hence the reason for Dr Langdon Down referring some of his doubtful patients to Professor Hutchinson. Syphilis, and therefore 'inherited' syphilis, like tuberculosis, was not an uncommon condition in those days.

Dr Sutherland and syphilis

Dr G. A. Sutherland was a well-known physician in his day and a frequently quoted authority on Down's syndrome. His description of the principal characteristics and aetiology of Down's syndrome, although written in 1900, is quite remarkable. His recognition and understanding of the pathology of Down's syndrome and also his observations of some of the attractive qualities to be found in people with Down's syndrome are little different from the way these things might have been sympathetically described fifty years later. However, in the light of the more positive views being expressed by the end of the nineteenth century, that syphilis as a primary cause was highly unlikely, Sutherland's view is eccentric. He is probably quite correct in saying, 'Some, starting in life the subjects of active syphilis, quickly waste and die,' but he went on to propose that Down's syndrome had its *origin* in syphilis.

The proposal that there was a causal link between syphilis and Down's syndrome was finally and totally rejected a few years after the turn of the century. It is highly unlikely that this suggested link has had much bearing on any prejudice against the mentally handicapped which might prevail today.

Alcoholism

Alcoholism, another condition which carries social stigma, has also been associated with Down's syndrome. Langdon Down himself suggested, in a paper published in 1887, that parental alcoholism may have had a part to play in the birth of a child with the syndrome, though the association between alcohol and mental handicap would seem to be much older. The notion that mental handicap was the result of a 'perpetual state of drunkenness', caused by the inability to 'digest a wine' already present in the child before birth, was referred to by Paracelsus in his writings of about 1530. Paracelsus is suggesting that all of us become drunk in the womb through the normal ingestion of alcohol which is taken by the mother, but most of us 'digest' it, coming to no harm. Those foetuses who are unable to accommodate the alcohol become mentally deficient. That, simply stated, was the theory.

His subsequent analogies are difficult to comprehend, being drawn as they were from contemporary theology. A more modern analogy would be that associated with drugs and the way a child can be born already addicted. Though Paracelsus went further by suggesting that the cause of mental handicap was not an *excessive* pre-natal intake of wine but a reasonably *normal* intake which was not properly 'digested'. He was not suggesting that the mother was an alcoholic. In this respect there is a difference from the drug addict who passes on the addiction. Perhaps Langdon Down's suggestion was a relic of this more ancient belief; though he did refer to alcoholism. Also the relationship between alcohol and sin, so much a part of the social conscience in the late nineteenth century, must have played a part; calling up the always present sense of sin being somehow linked with the birth of handicapped children as it had been since before the time of St Augustine. The idea that alcohol was involved in the cause of Down's syndrome was totally rejected by Sutherland in 1900.

It must be remembered that the characteristic features of Mongolism are present at birth, and they are of such a nature as to suggest a causative agent at work from a very early period of foetal life. General causes, such as alcoholism . . . are not likely to produce such an exact type of disease as exists in Mongolism.

Endocrine imbalance

From the 1920s onwards there was a good deal of discussion centred around the possibility that Down's syndrome resulted from an endocrine imbalance, either in the mother of the affected child or in the child itself. The endocrine glands produce hormones which are released directly into the blood circulation. The situation is exemplified by Clarke, who asserted in 1929 that 'every mongol has some endocrine imbalance'.

Maternal thyroid disfunction has probably been the focus of most discussion on this aspect, perhaps reflecting in some respects the Down's syndrome/cretinism confusion. Meyers, addressing the American Association of Mental Deficiency in 1938, related the occurrence of Down's syndrome to maternal hyperthyroidism. He told the conference about his observations of an 'acute nervous excitement' among his group of mothers of children with Down's syndrome and pointed out that many of them came from areas high in thyroid-related disorders. He concluded that maternal hyperthyroidism was the 'more prominent symptom of that peculiar but complex endocrine disturbance which is responsible for the occurrence of mongolism'.

Other researchers also noted the frequency with which thyroid disorders occur in mothers of children with Down's syndrome. Returning to Mantegna's *Madonna and Child* for a moment, it will be remembered that the speculation of the sitter being the child's natural mother arose from her obvious thyroid malfunction; possibly more of a coincidence than a causal relationship, unless the child was also suffering from hypothyroidism as well as Down's syndrome. This occurs with sufficient frequency for the dual problem not to be ruled out. It is interesting to note that maternal thyroid disease has been linked with an increased incidence of chromosome non-disjunction as recently as 1972.

The thyroid was not the only endocrine organ to be linked with Down's syndrome. Because some researchers found a delayed glycemic response (the presence of sugar in the blood), the pituitary was suspected. It was concluded by McDonald, as late as 1972, that 'hypofunction of the pituitary is an important factor in mongolism'.

Hypofunction of the thymus was also suspected of playing a part in the cause of Down's syndrome. One investigator reported 'gratifying results' when patients were treated with thymus gland. Sutherland, however, had dismissed this as a treatment in 1900 with the words '... treatment by thymus and thyroid extract has proved useless'. Similar kinds of claims have always been made for a variety of unconventional treatments, or even for the 'gratifying results' of treatments which appear to be reasonably orthodox but are later shown to be based on false or insubstantial theories; as was the case of treatment with thymus gland. It was most likely the extra care, attention and stimulation that these patients were receiving rather than the dose of thymus gland extraction which was responsible for the 'gratifying results'. Treatment of this kind, popular but mainly ineffective, will be taken up in a later chapter.

Reproductive system

Problems with the female reproductive system were from the earliest days considered to play a part in the birth of a child with Down's syndrome. One early suggestion was that a small amniotic sac prevented proper development. This problem is currently associated with successive miscarriages. Another theory was that diminished ova viability could explain many of the findings related to the aetiology of the syndrome. Yet another reported that young mothers of children with Down's syndrome often had a history of problems relating to fertility.

Increased maternal age and late position in the family were initially confused as factors contributing to an increased birth incidence of Down's syndrome, as some physicians had considered *both* maternal age and position in the family to be important factors. The correlation between maternal age and family size was obviously instrumental in this confusion, but maternal age was often rejected as a contributory factor because many cases of Down's syndrome were born to younger mothers. However, it is now widely accepted that maternal age *is* a most influential factor in the incidence of Down's syndrome.

In the late 1950s both maternal anoxia (lack of oxygen) and exposure to some form of radiation were noted as possible causes of Down's syndrome. Certainly the mutagenic effect of radiation had already been established for about twenty years. Mutation is normally a very infrequent event, though it can be greatly speeded up by irradiation with X-rays, gamma rays or neutrons. However, since there is mounting concern about the effects of radiation in the modern world, with nuclear explosions, nuclear power stations and all the attendant discussion which centres on this issue, the relationship between Down's syndrome and ionizing radiation will be dealt with separately.

When looking with hindsight at early reports and attempts to attribute factors causing Down's syndrome, it is all too easy to be dismissive about these efforts of the physicians and researchers of earlier times. But their concern with the truth and their dedicated struggle to solve the problems that presented themselves were surely no less creditable than the efforts of today's researchers.

CHAPTER 7

LIFE EXPECTANCY AND MAJOR DEFECTS

There can be no doubt about it, people with Down's syndrome are living longer. This must be attributable to better living conditions, better health care, more sophisticated surgical techniques and a more enlightened attitude to people with Down's syndrome. For example, they are becoming more involved in community life, sports and games, activities which make for maintaining and improving health. Table 3 gives a picture of this striking improvement in life expectancy.

It can be seen that an expectation of nine years in 1929 had increased four-fold in 1969, when the average life expectancy for people with Down's syndrome had increased to 36 years.

Beyond question the major cause of death in the past, as it is today, has been respiratory infection, with heart disease as a very close and associated second. The most frequent cause of death of children with Down's syndrome around the turn of the century was tuberculosis, as it was for so many others, especially children who were in any way delicate.

Table 3. Life expectancy [Adapted from Smith and Berg (1976)].

Place	Mean survival age	Year	Source
London, England	9	1929	Jenkins
London, England	9	1932	Penrose
London, England	12	1949	Penrose
Victoria, Australia	10	1954	Brothers and Jago
London, England	15	1958	Carter
Victoria, Australia	18	1963	Collman and Stoller
Surrey, England	35.5	1969	Richards and Sylvester
Mass., USA	32	1970	Fabia and Drolette
Texas, USA	30.5	1973	Deaton
Sheffield, England	40+	1985	Stratford and Steele

Conditions of life in the late Victorian era were not conducive to long life; infant mortality was high and survival into adulthood was not necessarily expected. In these circumstances, children with Down's syndrome would stand even less chance of long-term survival. Environmental pollution, unhygienic and insanitary conditions, infested and overcrowded housing and the consequent constant exposure to infectious diseases were at the root of high infant mortality, and children with Down's syndrome would suffer more than most. Immunization as a preventive measure against disease was still a thing of the future.

As living conditions, preventative measures and treatments have improved over the years, many common diseases have almost been eradicated and children with Down's syndrome have especially benefited from the improvements. Children with Down's syndrome have improved in health and increased in number as a result of better medical facilities and the elimination of once fatal diseases. The situation has resulted in one prominent physician describing the condition, not as a disease to be regretted but as 'part of our richer biological inheritance'.

However, even as the century progressed and things began to improve, children born with Down's syndrome continued to be sickly and early death was always to be expected. A study carried out by Carter between the years of 1944 and 1955, when infant mortality for 'normal' children was becoming exceptional, presents a pretty depressing picture for children with Down's syndrome. Carter surveyed the life spans of 725 children with Down's syndrome who were regularly attending the Hospital for Sick Children in London during those years. His subsequent data revealed that 60 per cent of these children were dead before the age of 10 years, 30 per cent of them dying before they were 4 weeks old. Carter was still, however, able to show an improving position. Dividing the period of his study into the years between 1944 and 1948 and between 1949 and 1955, he demonstrated that the mortality rate between the two periods had fallen by 40 per cent. A similar rate of improvement in life expectancy was also taking place in Australia at about the same period.

A quite dramatic improvement had occurred in 1970, when Fabia and Drolette published their life expectancy study in the USA.

They studied the prospects for 2,421 children born with Down's syndrome in Massachusetts in the year 1950. Ten years later, 67 per cent of boys and 62 per cent of girls were still living. Congenital heart disease had been the main cause of death in the early years for both boys and girls.

As Table 3 (page 53) shows, this kind of improvement has continued, though the critical years still remain the years of infancy and early childhood. Some limiting factors in the last three studies displayed in Table 3 account for what must seem to be very big increases in survival rates. Undoubtedly great improvements have been made in the intervening years, especially in heart surgery, both technically and in the skill and devotion of heart surgeons, though some discrepancy must still be allowed for in the two studies carried out in Surrey and Texas. Both these studies were conducted in institutions and consequently young children, i.e. those at higher risk, would have been too young to have been admitted. This condition is offset to some extent by the fact that statistics generally show that life span is not expected to be so great for those living in institutions as for those living at home. This is not a criticism of the quality of care exercised in institutions. It is simply that the more severely afflicted cases will be resident in institutions and their state of general health will tend to be more delicate. Deaton, who had conducted the Texas study in 1973, indicated that survival rates for individuals with Down's syndrome had been steadily improving during the previous twenty years. Of the original 1,018 Down's syndrome residents at the institution where the study was made, 927 were still living at the end of the ten-year period of the investigation.

The authors of the Sheffield study acknowledge that children under the age of 2 years were not registered on the records from which they drew their data, and of course these are the most critical years. Also, two mature gentlemen with Down's syndrome who had topped the age of 65 years slightly affected the averages!

During the 1960s and 1970s still more studies similar to those discussed above were conducted in different parts of Europe, particularly in Denmark and Sweden, and all the investigations reached the same conclusion: people with Down's syndrome were enjoying improved health and better prospects for a longer life.

Heart disease

Respiratory infections, resulting in pneumonia, are still the main cause of death in people with Down's syndrome, and this is especially true for infants and young children. However, some might be more inclined to point to cardiac defects as the principal cause of death, noting, as does heart surgeon Hallidie-Smith, that though chest infections amount to approximately the same number of deaths, '. . . it is conceivable that a congenital cardiac defect was a contributory factor in many of these patients'.

Just as antibiotics have reduced deaths from respiratory infections, so improved technical skills in heart surgery have reduced deaths from heart disease. Certainly heart surgeons are becoming confident and optimistic of success in performing operations on children with Down's syndrome. One Italian surgeon, working at the Vatican Children's Hospital in Rome, told me: 'If the child with Down's syndrome is 4 years old or less, the mortality rate should be no different from that of any other children, even though in Down's syndrome, the problems might be more severe.' It must be remembered, however, that although results continue to improve, the mortality rate for *all* children undergoing open heart surgery is still fairly high. Hallidie-Smith, and others offering figures, put the mortality rate at 20 per cent for children under 2 years of age and as high as 43 per cent 'even in centres of excellence' for infants under 3 months.

There is no doubt that the problem of congenital heart defects in Down's syndrome is still a cause for concern. There are an estimated 50 per cent of children with Down's syndrome so affected. This contrasts with less than 1 per cent in the population as a whole.

Most heart problems in children are those commonly called 'hole in the heart' (ventricular septral defect), and of all those children with heart disease, the distribution is about the same, at about 30 per cent for both children with Down's syndrome and others for this defect. The difference lies not just in the actual numbers but also with the more serious condition known as 'atroventricular canal defect', which is relatively rare in 'normal' children, accounting for less than 2 per cent of heart defects, though this serious malformation is present in about 60 per cent of children with Down's syndrome who have diagnosed heart disease. It is this latter malformation which is responsible for further complications, it being associated with the functioning of the lungs. This, of course, creates more problems of chest infections and associated respiratory difficulties.

A dilemma for cardiologists in their diagnosis and recommendations for surgical treatment of children with Down's syndrome is that many of these children are asymptomatic, that is, they are showing no distressing symptoms at the time of examination. If all things were equal there would usually be no hesitation on the part of the cardiologist to recommend early surgical intervention, taking into account the quality of life as the child grows up and passes the age of 40, when physical suffering is likely to become acute. In the not too distant past such a prognosis may not have caused too much conflict, but with the improving life-chances for people with Down's syndrome and their survival expectations now going well beyond the age of 40, the decision concerning early surgical intervention becomes more difficult to take.

Allowing for all the problems associated with heart defects and children with Down's syndrome, and without underestimating the seriousness of these conditions, the future promises well. Surgeons and those concerned with the medical management of these children are optimistic that the situation will continue to improve even further in the future.

Sensory defects

Of course, while visual defects and hearing difficulties are not in the same category of life-threatening seriousness as are heart defects, quality of life is important in the development of all children and that includes children with Down's syndrome. Sensory defects can have extremely serious implications for the all-round development of children, and these defects are over-represented in children with Down's syndrome. Perhaps deficiencies in vision and hearing have been responsible for many aspects of lack of progress in social and scholastic skills which have in the past been attributed to 'mental' deficiency. Happily these deficiencies are to a large extent remediable.

The eyes

The most outstanding physical characteristic in Down's syndrome is the archetypal shape of the eyes. It is this characteristic which led the early pioneers, Langdon Down, Fraser and Mitchell and those who immediately followed them, to ascribe and then to accept the label 'mongol' to describe those born with this condition. The epicanthic folds and narrow palpebral fissures (that is the fold of skin at the corner of the eyes and the apparently rather slanting, but narrow openings) were, until chromosomal karyotyping became possible after Lejeune's discovery in 1959, regarded as among the most characteristic and clear diagnostic signs of Down's syndrome in the newly born. Incidentally, oriental eyes only give the *impression* of being slanted due to more pronounced epicanthic folds which are absent in the majority of Europeans. These features, however, while affecting appearance, have no effect on vision. The feature is regarded by many as very attractive.

Another feature of the eyes of people with Down's syndrome is the presence of flecks of light colour in the iris, called 'Brushfield spots' after Dr Thomas Brushfield, the physician who first associated these features with Down's syndrome. While these light-coloured flecks (which incidentally give a 'sparkle' to the eyes) are present in the majority of children with Down's syndrome, they are also present in about 25 per cent of the 'normal' population. Again, this feature is purely diagnostic and has no effect on vision. However, *defects* in vision are characteristic features of Down's syndrome. Gardiner, a British opthalmologist, gave a figure exceeding 67 per cent of individuals with Down's syndrome having defective vision. The defects are either myopia (short sight, and possibly the most common defect), convergent or divergent strabismus (squint; though the epicanthic folds sometimes hide the presence of a squint from those who are not close to the affected child), astigmatism (the kind of elongated vision apparent in the paintings of El Greco, who was believed to suffer from astigmatism), or hypermetropia (long sight). All these conditions can be corrected by appropriate spectacles, though they need to be prescribed by a skilled optician who is knowledgeable and *interested* in children with Down's syndrome.

There are more serious eye defects associated with Down's syndrome, however. Blepharitis is a condition brought about by the dry and flaky skin which seems to trouble many people with Down's syndrome. The eyes become red and irritable and infections are easily attracted as a result of rubbing of the eyes to counter the irritation. This condition can be treated with prescribed ointments, but a first essential is keeping the eyes clean and removing any 'crusts' with warm water and cotton wool. Infections can cause corneal scars which can become permanent and even result in blindness if the offending infections remain untreated.

Cataracts are common in teenagers with Down's syndrome. There is a reported incidence of 50 per cent in patients with Down's syndrome, while such a condition is rare in an average population. Cataracts can be treated but need highly qualified specialist help. Cataract is a serious condition but especially so if left untreated. Blindness was discovered in just short of 10 per cent of patients with Down's syndrome over the age of 30 examined by Cullen in 1963. All the cases he examined resulted from cataract.

Opticians are becoming more aware of these eye problems associated with Down's syndrome. Modern approaches and methods are making things easier for more effective treatment to be offered and earlier diagnosis to be made.

Parents should not just seek an appointment with an optician but should question the optician very closely; if he/she appears to know little about Down's syndrome, they should shop around and find an optician who does.

The ears

Although abnormalities of the morphological structure of the ears have been noted in Down's syndrome, on the whole these children tend to have pretty little ears. They may be low-set and invariably there are very much reduced ear lobes. This is a feature which is also well represented in the 'normal' population, as many women who have difficulty in wearing earrings will recognize! While deformities in the *shape* of ears in Down's syndrome are comparatively rare, abnormal hearing is common. Hearing loss to a greater or lesser degree is frequently reported in children with Down's syndrome, the majority of problems arising from *otitis media*.

Otitis media is the middle ear problem which besets many children at about the age of 7 or 8. The problem with Down's syndrome is that the condition seems not to clear up spontaneously but to persist into adult life. Treatment for ear infections and the subsequent hearing loss is difficult to handle in patients with Down's syndrome, owing to the diminutive anatomical hearing mechanism. Surgical treatment including the insertion of grommets does not appear to produce good long-term results. Cleaning and syringing are effective, but only for a short time because the ears quickly become blocked again. However, modern hearing aids can be effective.

It is important to pay attention to hearing problems because good hearing ability can dramatically improve concentration and also improve the quality of speech and language development and consequently all other aspects of learning.

Other conditions

Down's syndrome, of course, does not offer protection and afford immunity from all the ills that beset the human race. Indeed, the person with Down's syndrome, as a result of poor natural immunity, tends to fall victim to any virus and infection which is 'going round'. Also their reaction to disease always seems to be more acute; they can be laid low by quite minor infections. This low level of resistance makes way for perpetual colds, unless special care is taken, since people with Down's syndrome are also quickly and extremely susceptible to extremes of temperature. Reduced sensory responses can cause further problems – the child with Down's syndrome will usually be less likely to seek necessary warmth or shelter.

There are some other conditions to which people with Down's syndrome are particularly prone, in addition to those afflictions such as heart disease and respiratory infections discussed above.

Alzheimer's disease

Alzheimer's disease, one of the age-old conditions of senile dementia, could also be called the disease of ageing. Its signs and symptoms are familiar in a number of old people: forgetfulness, unsteadiness, confusion, lack of orientation and consequent clumsiness, along with the general deterioration in faculties that often accompanies old age. Occasionally these symptoms of 'senility' appear earlier than might normally be expected. In these cases it is probable that the signs of early ageing are due to Alzheimer's disease. The early onset of Alzheimer's disease is common in people with Down's syndrome, particularly in those over the age of 40, (sometimes even earlier), though at the moment no one knows exactly when it might begin to show in the individual. It has been estimated that in the general population about 14 per cent of people aged 65 will show signs of dementia, yet Thase and his colleagues found that 45 per cent of patients with Down's syndrome had Alzheimer's disease from the age of 45, as against 5 per cent of other age-matched *mentally handicapped* people.

Not all are equally affected, but some of the signs can be recognized in most older people with Down's syndrome. This condition has become important in the medical management of Down's syndrome because of increased life expectancy. Of course, it was probably always present, though less noticeable, as the few people with Down's syndrome who lived to reach 'old age' would more than likely be in mental institutions where any dementia specific to Down's syndrome would hardly be differentiated from other patients in the institution. What is Alzheimer's disease?

Alzheimer's disease is a neuropathological (i.e. brain-related) condition which brings about changes in the features of the brain. It is a highly complex condition and a biochemical explanation along with morphological (i.e. anatomical and physiological) descriptions would be out of place here. Research is being carried out at the present time to find ways of curing, or at least ameliorating, the disease. The fact that it is so common in Down's syndrome means that scientists investigating Alzheimer's disease are involving more patients with Down's syndrome in their research. They may not be specifically interested in Down's syndrome but inevitably people with this condition will benefit from any results of their research.

Atlanto axial subluxation

Until the early 1970s, apart from a few minor irregularities, the spine was considered to be generally normal in people with Down's syndrome In the mid 1960s, however, a couple of investigators had noted a peculiar kind of spinal dislocation and speculated that this might result from some congenital abnormality. In recent years this particular weakness has become highlighted as a major problem for children with Down's syndrome and for those concerned with their physical development and socialization. It is now recognized that the problem known as 'atlanto axial subluxation', found in children with Down's syndrome (quite apart from being serious enough to cause total paralysis), can become a fatal defect if not carefully managed.

It appears that in this condition the top two spinal vertebrae are not properly aligned, and the peg-like piece of bone which links these vertebrae and also allows the spine to move freely is too short to be completely safe. The connection can easily become dislodged. Atlanto axial subluxation caused a good deal of alarm among officials involved in the 'Special Olympics' when the problem was raised at this relatively new international event. As a result of the subsequent publicity, consternation began to be felt all over the world; more and more youngsters with Down's syndrome were taking an active part in games and sports of all kinds, leaving them open to serious injury if this weakness happened to be present.

Fortunately the condition only affects about 2 per cent of the Down's syndrome population, though it should be said that it has been put at approximately 10 per cent at its highest. Even so, this is little consolation to those with Down's syndrome. For those engaged in sporting activities, or any other vigorous enterprise, it is like playing Russian roulette! In other words, who belongs to the small percentage with this problem? Its presence can quite easily be detected by X-ray, and it would certainly be advisable for all children with Down's syndrome to undergo this simple examination in order to discover those at risk and give peace of mind to the parents and guardians of the rest. Otherwise the whole of the population with Down's syndrome would have to refrain from some very enjoyable activities, even though more than 90 per cent of them would have no pathological need. The kind of pursuits to be avoided by the small percentage who are so afflicted would be: horse riding, diving, butterfly-stroke in swimming, football, high-jumping, gymnastics, trampolining, or any other activity which might put an undue strain on the spine. A protective collar can be fitted so that some activities can be undertaken by those children unfortunate enough to have this weakness.

Hepatitis

Since Blumberg reported in 1970 that people with Down's syndrome show a frequency of viral hepatitis ten times that of other mentally handicapped patients *in institutions,* there has been growing consternation about the consequences of this problem. To state his results briefly, Blumberg reported that in large mental institutions where viral hepatitis was endemic, all the residents with Down's syndrome suffered from a chronic type of hepatitis even though they showed no signs of jaundice. He accounted for this by drawing attention to the poor immune system in Down's syndrome and the unusually high representation of infective viral hepatitis in large institutions. In smaller mental institutions he found less, and among children with Down's syndrome living at home the number carrying the virus was almost negligible.

It would be irresponsible to ignore the dangers of a possible transmission of infection from a person carrying the hepatitis virus, but it is also reasonable to examine chances of this occurring. First of all, very few children with Down's syndrome who are living at home will in fact be carriers, but supposing that a few of them do carry the disease, it is the rate of *transmission* which must cause concern to those who are close to them. The risk must be very small indeed. Research which was carried out at the University of Nottingham revealed that teachers in special schools, who were in daily contact with children with Down's syndrome, numbered significantly fewer cases of viral hepatitis than could be expected in a random population of the same size from any source.

The problem with hepatitis is that after infection the antigen can be found in the blood for many years and repeated attacks are not unusual. This is especially true of affected children with Down's syndrome because of the faulty immune system.

Infrequent maladies

It is reported that the incidence of epilepsy is substantially less than might be expected in the general population, possibly occurring in less than 1 per cent of people with Down's syndrome. When epilepsy does occur, it is usually in conjunction with some traumatic event such as might happen to anyone else. In older adults (there is a reported increase in susceptibility in patients with Down's syndrome after the age of 35), epileptic fits, usually of the less serious kind, may result from the effects of Alzheimer's disease.

Also connected with Alzheimer's disease are a few reported cases of mental illness. Rollin, for example, writing in 1946, recounted symptoms of catatonic psychosis in patients with Down's syndrome, but it is highly likely, writing as a psychiatrist in a large mental institution as he was, that the behaviour he observed was either 'institutional' behaviour or was pathological in origin, due to Alzheimer's disease. Mental illness is very rare indeed in people with Down's syndrome. Perhaps the so-called normal population have something yet to learn from the demonstrably agreeable temper of people with Down's syndrome.

CHAPTER 8

THE EFFECTS OF RADIATION

Growing public awareness that ionizing radiation can have adverse effects on health has brought increased anxiety to different communities in many parts of the world. Disquiet has heightened as a result of radio and television discussions and reports, which raised disturbing issues because of indications that increasing doses of radiation from industrial sources might be responsible for an increased incidence of children born with genetic defects. A good deal of specific concern has been expressed regarding the possibility of a connection between radiation and any apparent increase in the birth of children with Down's syndrome. The suggestion of such a link is particularly disturbing to people living near nuclear power stations, or in areas high in natural radiation.

For example, a report in the *Guardian* of 11 November 1983 caused much uneasiness and became the subject of many subsequent debates. Frequently during these debates the main event was either forgotten or distorted. The basic facts of this event were that six babies with Down's syndrome were born to mothers who were teenagers together in a school in Dundalk (Ireland) when, it was reported, radioactive fallout from a fire at Windscale – 'Britain's worst nuclear accident' – reached the Irish coast. The fire had occurred in 1957 and '. . . the babies, two boys and four girls, were born between 1963 and 1972'.

Occurrences such as this might be coincidental, but it is natural, in the light of such events, that connections will always be sought, speculation will be made and fears will be voiced about the possible effects of ionizing radiation on the incidence of Down's syndrome.

It is important to remember that in Down's syndrome we are concerned with the induction of *chromosome* and not *gene* aberrations. Furthermore, Down's syndrome involves trisomy of 21, which is a numerical rather than a structural anomaly. Hence it is not the *breakdown* of chromosomes but the possible effect of radiation on the *number* of chromosomes that is of primary importance here.

The first work on the effects of radiation on chromosomes was carried out in the early 1920s, when James Watt Mavor investigated non-disjunction in the fruit fly *Drosophila melanogaster*, after exposure to X-rays. He found that X-rays caused the female to produce numbers of eggs with either no X chromosomes or with two X chromosomes, i.e. non-disjunction of the sex chromosomes. Later work by Patterson showed that the number of 'exceptional' (i.e. possessing an extra chromosome) flies produced could be increased by artificially ageing the eggs in the females before they were irradiated and mated.

However, these studies do not imply that X-rays are significant in the aetiology of Down's syndrome. There are two basic reasons for this:

(i)   The studies concern an extra X, not an extra 21, chromosome.
(ii) In the fruit fly there is no long dormant phase in the first meiotic division[1] in females as there is in humans or other mammals.

However, these investigations are important in that they were the first to indicate that non-disjunction could occur as a result of X-ray exposure. It is also notable that therapeutic doses of radiation to pregnant women had been suspected of producing congenital malformations as early as the 1920s. Consequently, once trisomy 21 had been identified, it is not surprising to find the aetiological significance of X-irradiation being questioned.

Investigations into medical X-ray exposure and birth incidence of Down's syndrome

The first survey which attempted to clarify the effect of X-ray exposure on the incidence of Down's syndrome was carried out in

1. The process of meiotic division is described and explained in the Appendix (page 160).

1959 by Lunn. He compared 117 mothers of children with Down's syndrome with the same number of age-matched mothers who did not have children with the syndrome. Both groups had received about the same degree of exposure to X-rays, and Lunn's findings showed no significant difference between these groups. Thus, according to Lunn, X-rays did not have any effect on the incidence of Down's syndrome.

Further studies followed and, in order to cover other possible effects and different types of malformation, some of the studies included a group described as 'sick controls'; that is, a group of mothers who had given birth to children with such defects as 'hare lip' or 'cleft palate', along with the more usual groups consisting of Down's syndrome births and 'normal' births. Unfortunately, all these studies and their results must be viewed with caution, because so many of them produced contradictory results. However, what is common to most of them is an apparent age-dependency effect. For example, it was recognized by the majority of the investigators that older mothers would have had a longer time to accumulate what would amount to 'heavy' irradiation exposure. A summary of the variable results from these experimenters is presented in Table 4.

One investigator, Sigler, examined the evidence of an association between leukaemia and Down's syndrome (children with Down's syndrome are more susceptible to leukaemia), together with the well-known and accepted relationship between radiation and leukaemia and the relationship between ionizing radiation and non-disjunction which had been demonstrated in laboratory animals. His hypothesis was that such associations gave reason to suspect a link between Down's syndrome and X-irradiation. Sigler and his colleagues compared the pre-birth X-ray exposure of a group of parents of children with Down's syndrome with a similar number of matched control parents. They found the following interesting significant differences between the mothers of the children with Down's syndrome and the controls:

(i)   17.7 per cent of 'Down's syndrome' mothers but only 8.1 per cent of controls had fluoroscopy prior to the birth of the index child. Within this group, the Down's syndrome mother tended to be older.

Table 4. Studies of medical X-rays and DS [adapted from Wald, Turner and Borges (1970)]. This table demonstrates the different results coming from separate studies of the effects of X-rays on Down's syndrome births and shows the lack of agreement.

Study	Location	Population	Results	Trends
Lunn (1959,	Scotland	117 DSM	NS	*
Uchida and Curtis (1961)	Canada	81 DSM	+	
Carter *et al.* (1961)	England	51 DSM	NS	‡
Stevenson and Matousek (1961)	Ireland	197 DSM	NS	*
Sigler *et al.* (1965)	USA	216 DSF	+	
Uchida *et al.* (1968)	Canada	861 M	+	
Marmol *et al.* (1969)	USA	61 DSM	NS	*
Stevenson *et al.* (1970)	England	1547 M	NS	*
Alberman *et al.* (1972)	England	489 DSF	+	
Cohen *et al.* (1977)	USA	216 DSF	NS	*

KEY
DSM Mothers of DS children
DSF Families with DS children
M   Mothers
NS   Not significant
+   Significant increase in DS births to exposed groups
*   Non-significant increase in DS births to exposed groups
‡   Non-significant decrease in DS births to exposed groups

(ii) 14.5 per cent of 'Down's syndrome' mothers but only 5.1 per cent of control mothers reported that they had received therapeutic exposure. Most of this extra radiation was for the treatment of skin conditions.

The doses in both these situations would tend to be higher than would be encountered in a single series of X-ray films for an isolated investigation (a broken limb for example). Sigler's interpretation of the results of his investigation was that 'mongolism is statistically associated with maternal radiation'. He also noted that this effect was not only accumulative, but that increased radiation sensitivity may contribute to the maternal age effect. Sigler concluded that X-rays may be involved in the pathogenesis (likely cause) of some cases of Down's syndrome.

However, despite the extremely thorough nature of this report, critics could still argue that the statistical association only reflects a general poorer health in the mothers of the children with Down's syndrome, since these therapeutic X-ray treatments were considered necessary. Further confusion is added by the findings of what was a virtual repeat of this study, the results of which showed no significant differences between cases and controls in respect of maternal X-ray history. All this shows how difficult it is to give a definitive answer to the apparently simple question: 'Will X-rays make the birth of a child with Down's syndrome more likely?' Also it shows that in highly complicated areas of human development containing many variables, the results of one, or even more than one, experimental study cannot be regarded as finally and totally reliable.

A balanced view which keeps things in better proportion comes from Alberman and his colleagues out of work they conducted in 1972. They speculated that a dose of 2,000 millirads (that is equal to about ten straight abdominal X-rays, or 360 chest X-rays) would be required to double the overall risk of Down's syndrome. They also pointed out that the effect of radiation alone would be very much smaller than the single effect of ageing, although the *combination* of both factors could be of some significance in the cause of Down's syndrome.

Overall, then, it seems that although there is some indication of an association between Down's syndrome and the amount of radiation received by mothers, we might say the question is not yet fully resolved.

Effects of other types of radiation

In terms of the whole world population, medical exposure to X-irradiation is equivalent to only one-fifth of the dose received from natural sources. This is not so surprising when it is remembered that the frequency of X-ray examinations in industrialized countries is ten times greater than in developing countries. Exposure to X-rays may well be the *major* source of radiation for those living in industrialized nations. If, then, this comparatively small amount can be of such consequence as to generate so much attention, the importance of considering other forms of radiation is all the more necessary.

Figure 2 shows the relative contributions of radiation from natural sources, nuclear power production, atomic explosions and medical exposures. While the contribution from nuclear power and atomic explosions is almost negligible (viewed in the context of the world population) when compared with natural sources, the doses received by the more closely exposed populations make them more likely to be of some significance.

(i) *Natural sources*

Included in this category are studies of geographical areas with high background radiation because of the natural rocks and ores. The type of exposure considered is typically that of a low dose 'per unit time' which occurs over a very long period of time.

A study carried out in New York in 1959 appears to be the earliest to mention Down's syndrome in this respect. The study considered congenital malformations in the context of the amount of background radioactivity involved. It covered more than 1.25 million live births in the period 1948–55, and it was revealed that in this period there were 16,369 reported babies born with a range of malformations. Geographical areas where the malformed births occurred were classified according to the existence of a 'probable' or an 'unlikely' presence of large quantities of radioactive rock or shale. The malformation rate was found to be significantly higher in the 'probable' areas than in the 'unlikely' areas. However, no significant differences were detected between the two areas for incidences of Down's syndrome. Consequently it was concluded that natural radiation was not linked with an increased incidence of Down's syndrome.

In the intervening years a number of different studies have been carried out, using a variety of methods, in attempts to establish any possible link between naturally occurring radiation and the birth of

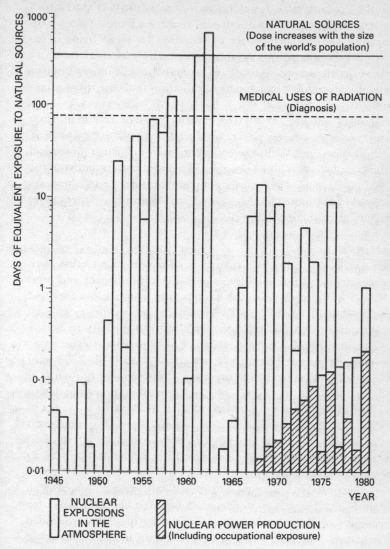

Figure 2. Comparison of exposures from different radiation sources. This graph shows trends with time of collective effective dose equivalent commitment per year of practice, expressed as days of equivalent exposure to natural sources [from United Nations publication (1982)].

children with Down's syndrome, but *none* of these has shown any clear correlation.

(ii) *Nuclear power production*
No specific investigations have been undertaken into the effects of *occupational* exposure of those workers involved in the nuclear industry and the subsequent birth incidence of Down's syndrome to these workers.

There is, however, one report following the incident in Ireland subsequent to an accident at the Windscale nuclear power station referred to earlier. In 1983, Sheehan and Hillary drew attention to an unusual cluster of births of infants with Down's syndrome to a group of mothers who attended a boarding school at Dundalk on the east coast of Ireland and were resident in the school during an influenza outbreak in October 1957.

The authors wrote that the accident to No. 1 pile at Windscale, which caused a fire releasing radioactive materials into the atmosphere, occurred at the same time as the influenza outbreak. This coincidence left them with 'nagging doubts' as to whether or not radiation, in conjunction with a viral infection, might affect non-disjunction. In their first report they published incidence figures for Down's syndrome in that area as reaching a level of 6 in 26 live births. This figure, however, represented the number of Down's syndrome births in a limited population and was abstracted from all mothers who had affected children. The study was not generally well received by the scientific community and came in for some severe criticism. At least four papers were written in 1984 pointing out its defects. Later, Sheehan and Hillary revised their figures to 1 in 24 by including the pregnancies of another 47 of the 213 children at the school in 1957.

While these researchers are open to criticism in the calculations of their statistics, there can be no dispute about the presence of the small cluster of Down's syndrome births. It may not be entirely reasonable to associate this cluster with the Windscale accident. Meteorological reports of the time show that, apart from a brief period of north-easterly travel, the radioactive cloud moved basically in a south-westerly direction, away from Ireland and over mainland UK and Europe. However, no increase in the incidence of Down's syndrome was subsequently reported in these regions. It would seem, therefore, that in spite of the unfortunate cluster of Down's syndrome births and the coincidental nuclear accident, there is no substantial evidence that the event had any effect on the rates of Down's syndrome birth incidences. At the same time, it is worth pointing out (as did Brown, one of the critics of the Sheehan account) that '. . . it would be logical to avoid any unnecessary exposure to possible mutagens that may add to the genetic burden of humans'.

A much more serious accident was that which occurred at Chernobyl in 1986. No reports have so far been made of increased incidences of Down's syndrome births, or unusual clusters of such births, resulting from the accident, but it is still early days. Mothers who give birth to children with Down's syndrome and who were unfortunate enough to be living within the reported fall-out zones are going to be difficult to convince that this accident was not concerned in any way with the birth of their children, whatever 'scientific' evidence may be presented in future analyses which might deny any connections. Many people, scientists included, will have 'nagging doubts'.

(iii) *Atomic explosions*
The survivors of the atomic explosions at Hiroshima and Nagasaki constitute a population that has been exposed to an extreme dose of radiation. Infants born between 1948 and 1954, whose mothers had been present in the cities at the time of the bombings, were examined. Only three cases of Down's syndrome occurred out of 5,579 births. The figures for this highly exposed population show an incidence of 1 in 1,860 Down's syndrome births; a great deal lower than the normally to be expected 1 in about 660. It could be considered that the huge doses of radiation encountered during these explosions would have caused an increase in gene and chromosome damage to such an extent that the spontaneous abortion rate would have escalated sharply. It could also have been assumed that such lethal mutations occurred more often among those women who might be more susceptible to non-disjunction. Also, of course, because of these devastating experiences, maternal physical and mental health may have been affected to such an extent that

miscarriages became more frequent. These factors would again be likely to select against any abnormal foetus. It should be noticed, however, that quite a number of *sex* chromosome trisomies have since been identified in children born to the survivors of these atomic bombings, but *no* autosomal trisomies have been identified.

Thus it is not realistic to compare the effects of such massive radiation doses with the smaller doses encountered during diagnostic and therapeutic X-rays or with even lesser doses resulting from natural sources.

Conclusions

While 'unusual clusters' of Down's syndrome births, which occur from time to time, will naturally cause disquiet in the communities where they occur, if those communities are near nuclear power stations or in areas high in radioactive rock, current scientific investigations of these circumstances seem to suggest that they are coincidental. At least there is no indisputable evidence that natural or accidental exposures have been directly responsible for such clusters or regional increases in birth incidences. With Down's syndrome constituting a common form of handicap in all parts of the world, it is likely that these apparently related events will occur from time to time, creating alarm and speculation.

Perhaps medical exposure to irradiation requires more explanation, in spite of, or possibly because of, conflicting, complicated and ambiguous reports.

The frequent diversion of opinion in reports concerned with the effects of X-irradiation could be interpreted as indicating that if the effect of X-rays is a factor in the incidence of Down's syndrome births, it is a very small factor. Perhaps X-irradiation *is* implicated in a few cases of Down's syndrome, and we might then justifiably ask what course of action, if any, should be taken. In the situation created by therapeutic radiation, the slightly increased risk of Down's syndrome cannot outweigh the risk from the disease being treated. X-rays are such useful diagnostic practices that eliminating or reducing their use would probably cause significantly increased risks to patients; this risk again overrides the possible increased risk of Down's syndrome in future pregnancies. It is perhaps also worth noting that ultra-sonography (sound scanning) often provides a suitable alternative to X-rays.

It is interesting to note that X-irradiation could perhaps be more clearly implicated in *supporting* the Down's syndrome population by virtue of its role in reducing the mortality rate of affected children. The assessment of heart defects, for instance, through cardiac catheterization and fluoroscopy, helps to prevent early deaths of many babies with Down's syndrome.

The continued thoughtful use of X-rays, together with an increase in the efficiency of X-ray equipment, should help to contain, if not reduce, any effects of the birth incidence of Down's syndrome. Hence it seems unlikely that X-irradiation, as a cause of non-disjunction, would promote any change in the prevalence of Down's syndrome.

CHAPTER 9

WHAT KIND OF TREATMENT?

Treatment

At the present time, there is no cure for Down's syndrome. Indeed, a cure, in the sense that we normally speak of 'cure', would always be impossible. The trisomy is involved in the constitution and very structure of the person with Down's syndrome. It is, however, more than likely that a 'cure' in terms of reversing or counteracting the effects of the extra chromosome will one day be found. This will depend on a more complete understanding of the biochemical reactions of the genes which are attached to chromosome 21, all of which have not yet been isolated. It is also exceedingly difficult to predict when this biochemical, genetic problem might be solved. Lejeune predicted, when I questioned him about the possibility, that such understanding will come within the next five years, though the general feeling in the scientific community is not so optimistic. The suggestion is that it may be well into the next century before such a 'breakthrough' in the field of cytogenetics could be made. The theory exists; turning the theory into reality is another matter, involving as it does highly complicated procedures and still many years' work in cytogenetic research. This future possibility does not help children with Down's syndrome who exist today, or those who will be born in the next few (or many) years. What can be done for them?

Naturally parents want to do all they can for their children, and parents of children with Down's syndrome are exposed to the siren song of every therapist who sounds the praises of their 'new' therapy, however unorthodox the treatment appears to be. Where is the parent who is going to deny their child any chance, remote or even outrageous though it might sound?

What is frequently not taken into account is that while Down's syndrome is a recognizable condition where all people with the syndrome have a similar karyotype, they are all equal in the way this extra chromosome affects them; there are many *individual* differences. Consequently each person needs to be treated according to the individual problems, medical, psychological, social, etc. which affect that person, quite regardless of the fact that they also have Down's syndrome. Of course, the person with Down's syndrome will be more likely to suffer from a greater number of afflictions than a person who does not have the condition, but they will be unlikely to suffer from *all* the ailments and problems which are associated with Down's syndrome as it is pathologically described, unless they are very unfortunate indeed.

The major defects associated with Down's syndrome and the treatments for these defects have already been discussed, but even accounting for these, by no means all children with Down's syndrome will be in need of such treatment. It was, for example, stated that about half the Down's syndrome population have serious heart defects; it must follow that the other half do not. It has also been pointed out that about 67 per cent of children with Down's syndrome suffer from some form of defective vision, and therefore it is essential that such children are given thorough ophthalmic testing. But it must also be clear that about 33 per cent of children with Down's syndrome do not have problems and have good average vision. The visual problems associated with Down's syndrome are particularly relevant in any discussion about individual differences, since the specific eye problems may be at opposite extremes – long sight, short sight, or a variety of other kinds of defect. It would of course be a great deal more convenient to announce that *all* children with Down's syndrome are shortsighted, for example, then universal advice could be offered to parents and opticians about short-sightedness in Down's syndrome. A tongue reduction operation can be performed on those children with Down's syndrome who have an inconveniently overenlarged tongue, but it would be absurd to perform the operation on those who do not suffer from having an enlarged tongue – macroglossia.

The same principle applies to other, less obvious, maladies. Consequently the medical treatment which might be extremely beneficial to one child with Down's syndrome may be of no benefit at all to another. Even worse, the treatment which benefits one child may cause some ill effects if administered to a child who does not need it.

The notion of generalized treatment possibly arises from the commonly held belief that 'mental' disability can be treated as a kind of separate 'mental/metabolic disorder'. Of course certain metabolic disorders which cause mental disability *can* be treated with medication, and it is perhaps because of these that confusion arises. Phenylketonuria (PKU) is one such disorder, Down's syndrome is not.

Plastic surgery

The most drastic treatment which is being offered to children with Down's syndrome is reconstructive surgery. Plastic surgery, a relatively new approach in the treatment of Down's syndrome, was first performed in Argentina in the mid 1970s; ten children were involved in this pioneering undertaking. The results were reported to other plastic surgeons at a meeting in Quito in 1977. A surgeon from Frankfurt named Hohler was sufficiently impressed to introduce the techniques within his hospital, operating in the same year on a girl with Down's syndrome whose nose was *extremely* flat and whose chin was *exceedingly* receding. The surgery did not make such a dramatic change in the child's appearance that she could not be identified as a little girl with Down's syndrome after the operation, but it was reported that she 'looked much less abnormal and underwent noticeable developmental changes'.

However, such reports must be regarded with caution. There are no objective criteria about what constitutes 'more' or 'less' abnormal appearance. There are even less objective measures for determining the effects of plastic surgery on 'developmental changes'. In spite of this and some ethical misgivings, a young plastic surgeon working at the time in Frankfurt was anxious to help children with Down's syndrome in any way he could. Gottfried Lemperle began a large series of operations on children with Down's syndrome. Lemperle's concern was to *improve* appearance rather than to bring about a complete and total change. This distinction is important in both ethical and social terms.

Who, for example, decides what constitutes a 'normal' appearance? There are, of course, conditions affecting appearance which put some people outside the wide parameters we think of as normal. An extreme example is a well-documented case of a South American child who was rescued by an eminent Scottish plastic surgeon. This surgeon restored the boy's face, building up and creating a nose where there had previously only been a hole. There are other abnormalities, e.g. cleft lip and palate (fortunately rare in Down's syndrome), for which surgery is required for cosmetic reasons but more essentially for the healthy survival of the individual. Few would dispute the validity of such surgery, but it is unreasonable to compare the case for cosmetic surgery in children with Down's syndrome with these conditions. It is also clear that some forms of simple cosmetic surgery are performed on children all the time, at the discretion of their parents, e.g. orthodontics (we don't think twice about seeking attention for misshapen teeth). Less common is surgery to correct outstanding ears and facial birthmarks. A fundamental difference, however, is that all these operations are performed indiscriminately for the whole population, not just for a particular sub-group to make that group less identifiable.

Tongue reduction for the over-enlarged tongue, present in some children with Down's syndrome, has been mentioned earlier; this is therapeutic and is cosmetic only incidentally. Lemperle certainly recognized this distinction, and of the sixty-seven children he operated on in Frankfurt between 1977 and 1978, tongue reduction was performed on sixty-three. The obvious significance of this particular surgery is the improvement in articulation reported by 68 per cent of parents of the children in Lemperle's 1980 study. It must be emphasized that this information has not been validated and is based on parental opinion, rather than the rigorous and objective criteria which would be built into a research model.

In view of the important implications of this form of surgery, there is urgent need for research into the precise articulatory changes brought about by tongue reduction surgery. Obvious benefit comes from the reported improved ability to close the mouth, similarly the increased area for resonance should improve vocal tone. By the time children reach the age of 4, however, some articulatory patterns are beginning to become established, and the child with Down's syndrome may experience difficulty in re-learning where to put the tongue to make correct sounds when he has a new tongue size; therefore the process of 'improvement' may be even slower and the results less dramatic. The need for reliable research into the effects on articulatory development is necessary to establish the exact nature and degree of improvement resulting from such surgery.

Parents naturally want what is best for their children and seek models from our society to know what that best is. They seek advice and opinions from professionals. At the Second International Down's Syndrome Congress held in Mexico City in 1983, a session on plastic surgery was interrupted by an Argentine mother who appealed: 'Don't ask me to change my child. I love her as she is.' This mother was speaking for the majority of parents all over the world. The pity is that parents of children with Down's syndrome are being put under pressure by society to believe that acceptance depends on their children undergoing a drastic change in physical appearance.

No reasonable argument can be put forward for changing the appearance of a child with Down's syndrome in order that the child becomes more acceptable to the society in which he lives. If society finds it difficult to accommodate the child with Down's syndrome, it is society which needs to change and not the child. Of course, such a change in attitude is difficult to bring about. It is a great deal easier to change the minority to suit the likes and dislikes of the majority, but the majority are not always right. George Bernard Shaw's maxim for the revolutionist was: 'The reasonable man adapts himself to the world: the unreasonable man persists in trying to adapt the world to himself. Therefore, all real progress depends on the unreasonable man.'

Metabolic disorders

A number of reports have appeared in the literature addressed to the problems of biochemical abnormalities in Down's syndrome. The abnormalities are quantitative rather than qualitative and are therefore less easy to investigate. Growth patterns in Down's syndrome, for example, are not typical of the 'normal' population.

There is significant retardation in both weight and height. Disorders in protein, carbohydrate and fat metabolism, as well as mineral and vitamin deficiencies, have been found. These show themselves as variations in serum globulin components, glucose tolerance, and cholesterol, electrolyte, and calcium levels. Vitamin A and B metabolism also appears to be altered. Children with Down's syndrome may also have a high incidence of gastro-intestinal tract disorders and especially a problem of poor absorption of essential nutrients, all of which can affect growth.

However, whenever well-controlled studies have been carried out on growth patterns, findings have not differed significantly from what might also be found within the normal range. The reasons for specific investigations into protein metabolism, for example, have been on account of the increased susceptibility to infections. Abnormalities in glucose tolerance have also been noted, and an impaired gastrointestinal absorption has been suggested as a possible reason for this.

Vitamins

A study of various metabolisms has led investigators to consider the possibility of disturbed vitamin B_6 in the bodily chemical process in Down's syndrome. Investigators have suggested that children with Down's syndrome easily become more deficient in vitamin B_6 than do others because (a) there appear to be lower stores of this vitamin in the body, (b) there is an increased rate of excretion of the end product of the chemical process. However, this kind of study is like many others: it only needs to be proposed, to be in another situation denied by other studies which have taken into account other variables. For example, one study which carefully examined the proposed B_6 disturbance in children with Down's syndrome also examined their brothers and sisters, finding no differences between them and their Down's sibling; thus indicating that the supposed deficiency had less to do with Down's syndrome than with the environment where the subjects of the experiment were living.

Consistent results of investigations concerned with metabolisms have rarely been obtained. In fact there are many studies which indicate no more disturbance in Down's syndrome than can be found in the 'normal' population as there are studies which find differences. Given the wide range of reactions and susceptibility to disease of children with Down's syndrome, this is hardly surprising. Of course, it must be repeated that metabolic problems *can* be present in Down's syndrome which will need to be treated. The treatment, however, is no different from the treatment which would be given to anyone else. Such problems are not exclusive to Down's syndrome.

Nutrition

Although, on the basis of current knowledge, nutrition appears to play no part in the aetiology of Down's syndrome, the deviations in growth, biochemical differences and feeding problems emphasize the importance of nutrition in the management of children with the condition.

As a result of the general delay in the rate of growth, the appearance of oral reflexes is frequently delayed in Down's syndrome. In addition, the social skill of self-feeding is retarded. All the usual and normal progressions from baby food to regular eating will be later. The problems have been summarized as follows:

(i) For the young infant, there will usually be a poor sucking habit and a difficulty in swallowing.

(ii) Sometimes the tongue will be enlarged and 'drooling' will result. There will often be poor lip and tongue control.

(iii) Malalignment of the jaws and a tendency to thrust the tongue forward may cause a delay in accepting solid food.

(iv) A delayed appearance of the chewing reflex and later eruption of teeth is associated with difficulty in chewing.

(v) Difficulty in swallowing may be due to xerostomia (dry mouth) where there is a decreased production of saliva.

There is no adequate synthetic substitute for food and correct eating habits. Basically, anyone who has a balanced diet does not need to take vitamins. While nutritional requirements may vary in different parts of the world, in Britain it means including four basic food groups in what we eat, and this is equally true for children with Down's syndrome, unless of course there is some other *specific* problem present in the child's constitution. The four main constituents of diet should be bread and cereals; fresh fruit and vegetables; meat (including fish and poultry) or meat substitutes in the case of vegetarians, which would include beans and lentils, soya and eggs; and finally the milk group which includes dairy products containing milk, such as cheese.

Tablets and pills can never be a substitute for proper food. Manufactured chemicals can never supply *all* that the body needs to function properly. In fact, scientifically speaking there is much which is still unknown about the precise composition of food. Food is always richer than any vitamin supplement could ever be. Of course, one problem with children with Down's syndrome is that they seem to acquire a taste for the 'wrong' things, so they become prone to obesity and other problems concerned with eating 'not wisely, but too well'. Some confusion also arises because there is always the possibility that the obesity in children with Down's syndrome *may* have its origins in a metabolic disorder of some kind.

It is *balance* more than amount which needs to be maintained. But even though we all tend to eat less than perfectly, real vitamin deficiencies are rare these days. Doctors are becoming more reluctant to prescribe vitamins except in cases where a patient is unable to eat, or has for example a low haemoglobin level where iron supplement would be required, or some other well-recognized metabolic condition – Down's syndrome is not one of them.

Water soluble vitamins (B and C) are easily passed out of the system and do little harm, but the fat-soluble vitamins (A, D, E and K), being stored in the lipids, are much more difficult to remove than the water soluble ones. The dangers involved in taking these to excess cannot be ignored. A build-up of any one of them creates adverse toxic effects in the system. At the extreme it can result in what has been called 'polar-bear's disease'; this is so named because polar bears carry such an excessive amount of these vitamins that their livers are poisonous to the human system.

The safest attitude that any parent of a child with Down's syndrome can take, for the child and for themselves, is never to indulge in vitamin treatment on a do-it-yourself basis. *Always* seek advice from those who are medically qualified and able to give the right kind of advice.

Management

The major objectives for dietary management in Down's syndrome should include:

(a)   The promotion of self-feeding skills.
(b)   The avoidance of obesity by including the right kinds of food.
(c)   The prevention (or correction) of any nutritional deficiencies which might develop as a result of the earlier mentioned biochemical abnormalities.

Effects of vitamins on intelligence

A sensational report by Harrell and her colleagues in 1981 generated considerable interest in the scientific community and in the popular press, when significant gains in I Q were highlighted in children with Down's syndrome following a course of treatment by megadose vitamin supplements. Unfortunately, the methodology and analysis did not stand up to scrutiny. It must be emphasized that Ruth Harrell was concerned to help children with Down's syndrome and genuinely believed that her approach had helped. She was not aware that some of the scientific short-cuts which had been taken would invalidate the results. However, scientists were sufficiently alerted to replicate her proposed treatment while at the same time controlling the variables which had been out of control in the Harrell study. The first to report the results of a replication study was Caislin Weathers in 1983. Using exactly the same megadose formulae, she reported:

In a double-blind study, 24 Down's syndrome children, ages 7–17 years, living at home, were given a megadose multi-vitamin supplement for four months [i.e. the same time as was given in the Harrell study]. A matched group of 23 children received a placebo in identical form. The children's I Q, vision, and visual-motor integration were tested before and after supplementation, and weekly checks were made to monitor behavioural changes. *No differences were found between the two groups on any measure as a result of supplementation* (my italics).

Undeterred, possibly as a result of popular pressure to investigate further, a much more extensive study was conducted in the United States under the direction of Professor George F. Smith, a leading authority in the field of Down's syndrome. He and his team followed a much bigger sample over a longer time and with more variables. Their conclusions were similar to those of Caislin Weathers except that '. . . both groups showed a comparable amount of improvement with no difference between the two groups'. This of course indicates that attention and care are the most effective 'techniques' for improvement.

There is an important message, which is relevant to all research, in a report of the Smith study which reads: 'Each hypothesis must be subjected to careful clinical study before instituting treatments which may at the least lead to disappointment and dashed expectations, and at the worst to harm for those children we are so anxious to help.'

Dr Sigfried Pueschel, one of the leading medical authorities in Down's syndrome today, has stated quite categorically that he considers nutritional intervention to be 'pointless' as a means of improving intelligence.

Gland and cell therapy

While something might be said for the advantages of vitamin therapy, especially if properly prescribed when deficiencies are diagnosed, nothing can be said for the so-called cell therapy.

The first attempts at this kind of treatment were made at the turn of the century and were even then dismissed. Sutherland, writing in the *Lancet* of 1900, wrote:

It is stated by some authorities that thyroid gland treatment has a beneficial effect in Mongolism, but such has not been my experience. I have given it a prolonged trial in four cases and with the exception of *a loss of weight and a rise in temperature*, no perceptive change in the condition was effected. A similar result has followed from the employment of thymus gland. Two patients aged respectively seventeen and fourteen months have been treated with thymus gland in increasing doses, and at the end of six months no alteration in the general condition could be detected. (My italics.)

Besides various kinds of enzyme, hormone or tissue therapies, there is also the so-called cellular therapy or Niehaus therapy, called after the Swiss surgeon who first put it into practice in the 1930s. It is this particular cell therapy which, according to the advocates, is the choice for Down's syndrome.

Dried cells, coming from the foetuses of the black sheep, are prepared for the treatment of children with Down's syndrome. These preparations contain practically all the normal cell constituents such as nucleic acids, histones, enzymes, protein, etc. What is the scientific basis for this treatment?

The scientific basis

The Belgian geneticist Van den Berghe has summarized the scientific basis for cell therapy and has divided it into three categories. Firstly, there are papers which are highly unscientific. These are often well supported by uncontrollable case reports and statements about the therapeutic activity of the treatment. These therapies are not experimentally verified, are untestable and are thus worthless hypotheses. The second category are papers containing a good deal of well established scientific information from other sources but this information is included very partially, sometimes in the introduction and sometimes in the discussion. The data, however, is not related to the established evidence and the citations are irrelevant. Sometimes the information is presented in such a way that it covers what is subtly or overtly false.

There are some papers, however, which do meet the criteria for scientific quality. It is these which constitute the scientific basis for the theory because these articles are cited whenever 'the ultimate proof' is called for. According to the theory, cell therapy is activated by stimulating corresponding organs, for example heart cells stimulate the heart, liver cells stimulate the liver. There is still no valid scientific basis for this belief. However, let us ignore the scientific basis; if the administration of whatever cell preparation would result in a cure or a considerable improvement in the physical or intellectual function of children with Down's syndrome we would be delighted to prescribe it. Like the early treatment for pernicious anaemia, we would be ready to eat raw liver, or raw cells, if it would help. Unfortunately, as Van den Berghe has noted, 'Thirty years of cell therapy in Down's syndrome during which thousands of these children have been treated, have not given any convincing evidence of effectiveness.' Who then would consider this to be beneficial to a child with Down's syndrome when we know all too well how much more sensitive the child is to infection than normal children?

Years ago there was a possibility of infection by zoonoses (diseases communicated from animals to man), and instances are known of fatal infections. At the present time, however, the cell preparations are quite safe in this respect. Even so, there is always a possibility of autoimmune manifestations because antibodies against certain animal organs cross-react with human organs. There has been no long-term follow-up of children who have been exposed to this kind of treatment, though it appears that major accidents occur very infrequently.

CHAPTER 10

COUNSELLING

Genetic counselling

It is well known that Down's syndrome occurs at a fairly constant rate in all parts of the world at somewhere between 1:600 to 1:700 live births. However, this ratio is not evenly distributed among females within child-bearing ages. It is equally well known that the possibility of having a child with Down's syndrome is age-related. Simply stated, this means that it is more likely to occur in older mothers than in younger mothers, though there is some more recent evidence suggesting that very young mothers also stand at greater risk. Generally speaking, the chances fall into the following age categories: at the age of 20 the chance would be 1:2,000, at 30 it would be 1:1,000, at 35 the chances are only slightly more than the 1:660 generally quoted average, being about 1:500; only later do the chances increase steeply to 1:80 at age 40 and to 1:17 at age 45. It must, however, again be pointed out that the majority of children with Down's syndrome are in fact born to mothers in the 20–29 years age range, which is simply because the majority of babies are born to mothers in this age range. About 65 per cent of all babies with Down's syndrome are born to mothers in this age group.

More than 95 per cent of Down's syndrome births are the uncomplicated trisomy 21. The extra chromosome is attached to, and similar to, the 21st pair. Mothers who have given birth to a child with Down's syndrome will ask sooner or later what the chances are of having a second baby with Down's syndrome. The answer to this question is quite straightforward; there is a slightly increased chance, but this increased chance is almost negligible. In 'common' terms it can be assumed that the chances for a particular mother are just the same as they were previous to this birth and to the general female population, that is any other female within the same age group. So if the mother is, say, 22 years old when she gives birth to a child with Down's syndrome, her chances of giving birth to a second child with Down's syndrome still remain at about 1 in 2,000. However, if she is over 40 and under 45 years of age, allowing for the fact that her chances of conceiving any child will be less, her chances are still high, but no more than they were before – around 1 in 80.

As was stated previously, these figures account for around 95 per cent of Down's syndrome births. The remaining figure of approximately 5 per cent has to be considered.

It has been estimated that this 5 per cent (4.7 per cent to be statistically precise) of Down's syndrome births will be translocation (see Appendix for a full description and explanation of translocation). This is a chromosome arrangement where the extra number 21 chromosome is not attached to the other pair but is located (i.e. translocated) on another pair, in another group, which could be either number 13, 14 or 15. The specific number or group is of little account, except to geneticists. The translocation results in no obvious observable difference in the child, either in appearance or development, from that of any other child with Down's syndrome.

However, the significant feature is that this translocation type of Down's syndrome will most likely occur because the mother is a carrier. While the mother will have a normal complement of 46 chromosomes and will be in all respects perfectly normal, one of her pair of 21 chromosomes will be attached to another group, in other words instead of there being a pair of chromosomes on 21, there will be only one, the other being attached to 13, 14 or 15. This mother's chance of having another child with Down's syndrome will be significantly increased, to 1 in 5. This translocation is fortunately very rare. Even rarer is another type of translocation; this is a type which can occur within the same chromosome size group, that is from 21 to 22 in the G group. The genetic principle is the same for both mother and child, but in this very rare condition the difference is that *every* live birth would be Down's syndrome.

Transmission – implications for parents and siblings

Following the birth and subsequent settling down period and acceptance of a baby with Down's syndrome in the family, parents
frequently ask about the implications of the birth of a child with
Down's syndrome for their family; themselves as possible parents
of future children and the baby's siblings as potential parents. At
this stage they are less concerned with the emotional and stress
factors which result from the child's presence in the family; they
are most frequently concerned about the genetic factor. Is this
condition hereditary? Can it be passed on?

The following incident is typical of this concern, though expressed from a slightly different perspective. A young man tele-
phoned recently; he was shortly to be married and his fiancée had a
sister with Down's syndrome. He put his question with great embarrassment and mentioned the shame he felt in putting it, but said
that he really needed to know what the chances were of his future
wife 'inheriting' the condition. He need have felt no shame, the
question is a reasonable one to put, because a number of genetic
anomalies are due to recessive genes and as such are inherited.
However, this is not the case in Down's syndrome, which is not
caused by recessive genes. There is no more chance of a brother, or
a sister, or a cousin of a person with Down's syndrome having a
child with this condition than there is for anyone else *in the same
age group*. Any relative of a person with Down's syndrome who
does have a child with Down's syndrome can be assured that the
birth has occurred coincidentally. After all, with the birth incidence
rate at around 1:660 such 'coincidences' are bound to occur.

Pre-natal diagnosis

There are techniques by which the development of Down's syndrome can be detected in the early stages of pregnancy. The most
common of these techniques is a test known as amniocentesis.
Some time between fourteen and sixteen weeks of embryonic development some of the fluid can be drawn from the amniotic sac in
which the baby is developing. At this time the cells of the baby will
be present in the fluid and it is possible then to examine these cells

to discover whether the extra chromosome, indicating Down's syndrome, is present. This treatment is not, however, freely available to every woman who is pregnant. Quite apart from the cost to the health service, it would not be wise to apply this technique without good cause. Though such incidences are rare, there is always the possibility of the procedures involved in carrying out an amniocentesis harming a perfectly healthy foetus or perhaps inducing a spontaneous abortion. At the present time amniocentesis is more likely to be offered, or made available, to pregnant women over the age of 35, or to those who are considered to be 'at risk'. It is not so easy to determine or to decide who might be classified as being 'at risk', particularly among younger mothers; any mother who was a known carrier would be an obvious case.

Some indications of the likelihood of a Down's syndrome pregnancy can be obtained by taking a blood sample from the mother; this can be taken much earlier in the pregnancy. There is no certain identification from the blood test results, but they can provide evidence to indicate that amniocentesis might be advisable. This evidence would be a low level of alphafetoprotein (AFP); there tend to be lower levels of AFP (a chemical substance) if the pregnancy is one of Down's syndrome. Low levels can suggest a Down's syndrome development, but on the other hand low levels of AFP can also be found in the blood of mothers who are carrying normal babies.

A newer, potentially safer (depending on skill) and in many ways more effective technique for pre-natal diagnosis is one known as chorionic villi sampling. This technique was originally investigated in 1969 but was not developed until around 1975 when the Chinese used it for sex determination. It was not until 1983 that it was sufficiently well developed for use in karyotyping. Italian research workers were the first to diagnose Down's syndrome by chorionic villi sampling. A sample (biopsy) is taken by passing a catheter attached to a syringe into the uterus; this is guided by an ultra sound scanner. The single great advantage of this method, apart from the possible safety factor, is that a reliable diagnosis can be made as early as the eighth week of pregnancy.

Pre-natal diagnosis is a controversial issue. Opposing views are taken as to the necessity or desirability of the examination.

Some parents who believe they may be 'at risk' will wish to have the diagnosis in order that their anxieties may be allayed, or that they may consider the options open to them should their anxieties be justified – that their baby is handicapped. They may decide to request an abortion, or to use the information acquired, spending the intervening period before the birth adjusting to different expectations and preparing from the earliest days for the problems and difficulties which will inevitably be encountered.

Other parents will see no necessity and have no desire for pre-natal diagnosis. Their moral convictions about the sanctity of life would make abortion out of the question, even if it was revealed to them that their child was handicapped.

A small number of parents might request pre-natal diagnosis for other reasons, not having thoroughly considered the full implications. These parents will need sensitive counselling, preferably before the diagnosis is undertaken and most certainly afterwards if it does indicate that the baby is handicapped.

The availability of pre-natal diagnosis is bound to cause a dilemma for both parents, but perhaps more particularly for the mother. It is one thing to learn very early in pregnancy that a baby with Down's syndrome has been conceived who is as yet a completely unknown child, and quite another to have learnt to love the child as a living human being, growing and developing, whose small achievements can bring such relatively large rewards. Maybe to the mother the baby has always been human in a special kind of way, which is why I say the dilemma is more poignant for her than for the father. One mother I know spoke for so many when she said that had she known she had been carrying a child with Down's syndrome she would have had no hesitation in seeking an abortion, but she went on then to say how pleased she was that she had not known:

There is no way I would swap Angela for a 'normal' baby, she is more loveable and worthwhile the way she is. She is leading a full, reasonably self-sufficient life and I wouldn't have it any other way. Yes, we've had our problems, but what child doesn't cause problems?

And another mother who told me:

Of course, for herself you know, I'd like her to be normal, but for me, and my husband as well, we love her as she is; in fact we wouldn't want to change her for a 'normal' baby even if we could. Maybe parents who don't have a baby with Down's syndrome wouldn't understand that but it's true. Thank God I didn't know till after she was born or I might have had an abortion and I would have lost so much more than a baby – if you understand my meaning.

Breaking the news

Much professional concern centres on the issue of timing in this sensitive matter. When should the parents be told that their new baby has Down's syndrome and who should be the person to tell them?

Research by Janet Carr seems to suggest that the majority of mothers want to know as early as possible. All would agree that the information should not be withheld from parents should they inquire about handicap. Even if the position is not quite clear, parents have the right to be kept as fully informed as they wish to be in these circumstances.

There is extensive literature concerned with informing parents of the diagnosis of severe mental or physical impairment in their child. Despite the range of opinions to be found in the literature, no one clearly 'preferred' time has been identified as the optimum time for imparting the news. There is still considerable difference of opinion as to the point in time at which parents should be told that their child is handicapped, should this telling be necessary – many parents come to the realization from their own observations. Several studies have considered this time as one of crisis, producing immediate grief, followed by stages of shock, disbelief, denial and anger, later resolving into adaptation and adjustment – these phases are similar to those identified in the literature on bereavement. It has been suggested that the way in which parents are told of their child's impairment is critical, and may well affect the way in which they adjust to the situation and their early treatment of the child.

Parents frequently report dissatisfaction with the way in which they were first informed of their child's handicap and at the lack of sensitivity displayed by the professional imparting the news, whether doctor, midwife, paediatrician or psychologist. Giving such news must always be one of the more unpleasant tasks these professionals have to perform. Sometimes it is a question of unease which creates the difficulty for the professional concerned, and they may sincerely believe that the news should be broken quickly and unequivocally; this belief, combined with their own feelings of embarrassment and helplessness, too often results in an abrupt, apparently unconcerned disclosure of the news. At this stage the professionals may feel that there is little else to add to the diagnosis, since the prognosis may not be very clear. Questions raised by parents may be outside the experience of the professional concerned, who may also consider them not relevant *at that time*. This situation tends to give the professional a sense of insecurity, which in turn is conveyed to the parents.

Most parents want to know as much as possible about the condition and prognosis from the very beginning, yet it is generally recognized that they cannot cope with too much information at one time. Time is needed to consider and discuss the same facts many times before they can grasp their full significance.

Much of the dissatisfaction reported stems from the timing of the first diagnosis and identification of mental handicap. In a study directed specifically at parents of children with Down's syndrome who reported dissatisfaction on this point, the following points were noted. There was delay and evasion before the diagnosis was made known; sometimes there was initial denial; babies were taken away from the mothers immediately after birth, and no explanations were offered for their removal; they were put in special care nurseries without explanation; nursing staff behaved 'oddly' towards the mothers; the mothers' questions were evaded or ignored. While it was frequently noted that the time interval between a mother's expressed suspicion and a definite diagnosis being made was comparatively short, it was still sufficient to raise parental anxiety and anger.

It was apparent from the comments in this study, conducted quite recently by Quine, that most would have preferred to have been told that something might be wrong as soon as possible (as would the mothers in Janet Carr's study), even if the doctors might still be uncertain as to the exact nature of the impairment. Any delay and uncertainty were reported as having led to additional distress for parents, and in some instances may have been responsible for deteriorating relationships between parents and doctors. There are many ways in which these encounters can go wrong. The doctor may feel that he or she has been both sympathetic and informative and then be dismayed when, at their next meeting, parents seem to remember little of what they have been told; sometimes this dismay turns into annoyance. Perhaps the professionals do not always appreciate that parents, however calm they may appear, may be experiencing severe shock and anger at the moment of receiving the news; clearly these feelings can affect the way in which they are able to receive the information. Since the way in which the news is imparted to parents is known to affect the level of trust and respect in subsequent encounters with professionals, it is important that this issue is handled with great care. At this level there is concern about the encounter between *individuals*, at another level there is a need for professionals to give consideration to the broader structural context in which the encounter takes place.

For many parents the initial diagnosis is likely to come as a severe blow, confirming their worst fears. It removes any hope that the fears they have been experiencing are groundless, but rather makes it clear that the problem is more permanent, that it is not just a temporary complication, removable by medication or minor surgery. Instead it will involve the family in radical re-thinking, in consideration of long-term adjustments and implications.

Some parents may experience feelings of relief that at last the uncertainties, doubts and nameless fears are resolved; the known can be dealt with, the unknown is stressful. Diagnosis has clarified the position, the 'worst' is known. Now they can come to terms with the problems and can face them in their own way and in their own time.

After the diagnosis

A self-evident truth is that *parents are people*; their reactions to stressful situations will be many and varied, according to their personalities, previous experiences and general ability to cope. What does seem to be common to most parents is an inability to process and absorb the amount of information they request very soon after being told of their child's handicap. The immediate shock of the initial diagnosis tends to reduce the capacity to remember what they are being told. Questions are asked and answered but answers may not be heard or, rather, registered. Information is offered, but not always processed in the parents' minds.

Questions crowd into parents' minds but which questions should they ask? The most basic ones can be easily and positively answered: 'Will she walk? Will she talk?' The answer is 'Yes, perhaps a little later than normal, but yes.' Other questions can cover anything which is of immediate concern, but the professional must be prepared to answer the same questions many times. In order to give parents time to adjust to the first shock, some time needs to be allowed. Not too long or the parents will feel abandoned. Medically, there is very little a doctor can do at this stage and the temptation is to make an appointment too far ahead. I believe that *both* parents should be seen together within two to three weeks of the first diagnosis, and then again shortly after. Questions will become more rational, and information relevant to the parents' needs and circumstances gradually absorbed. They may not wish to *know* about human genetics, let alone understand it, so this aspect should be left until there is an indication that such biological information is wanted. Early contact can be made with the Down's Syndrome Association, who will help in any way necessary, later offering relevant literature.

For the professional, implications are that these early questions *need* to be answered, but must be answered in a simple, straightforward manner. There is time enough later for parents to ask again, and learn more detail, about the condition. Perhaps an assurance of further opportunities to meet with other professionals involved in the field of Down's syndrome would help to reduce anxieties in the first meetings and provide reassurance for the longer term that professional involvement will not end at this stage.

The first essential, for the professional, is to work towards helping the parents to come to terms with the implications of the diagnosis and at some level to accept their new baby. More often than not, when faced with a tiny, helpless and usually appealing baby, the parents have little difficulty in accepting it. At all costs the professionals should not themselves obstruct or hinder this acceptance. The following letter from a young father describes a situation which is not untypical.

Jason was born on the 11th April 1985. He was our first born and looked perfectly O K, and why shouldn't he. My wife was only 21 years old and me 26 years old. She had a perfectly normal pregnancy and a very easy birth. He was 6lb 12oz and had his eyes wide open the minute he was born and looked absolutely beautiful.

The morning after he was born my wife was informed he was very floppy and they were going to take a blood test to find out why. That was a Friday morning and we were told the results would be back by the evening. Eventually after a lot of persisting from us to find out if the tests were back, we were told we would have to wait till Monday because everyone had gone home for the weekend. Finally at 6.00 p.m. on the Monday, my wife and I were told that Jason had Down's syndrome; on hearing this, which at the time was a shock, it knocked us for six.

We had a long talk from the paediatrician, but I must add that at the time her words seemed to just pass through us. My wife immediately decided she wanted to go home with me and the baby, we then had another 3 hours wait while doctors and nurses tried to talk her out of it. Jason hadn't been feeding very well, to which I must add my wife never got any help or advice about. She was put in a room on her own with the baby, and left to it, so the doctor that night was trying to tell her that it wasn't advisable to leave the hospital until he was feeding O K, then my wife said all right she would leave him there until he was feeding better and *she* would go home. The doctor's first reaction was 'You can't do that, you may decide not to come back for him!' My wife, who was outraged at that, said, 'Fair enough, I'll take him home tonight!' So eventually he decided that he would let us go.

For about 2 weeks I felt as if I had lost something and that the world was against us and that nothing would ever be right again. But now 2 years on and with another addition, Richard, who is just under a year younger, my wife and I have had more pleasure out of the 2 boys than can be put on paper. Just to watch them together is a joy, they sit and play together and what one does the other will copy. Neither can walk yet but they have both just started to be daring and let go when they are standing. There is not much Jason can't do except for walking. He has just started to say one or two things and is beginning to pick up a few Makaton signs, he knows everything you say to him, because if you ask him to do something or not do something he'll do exactly what you say. He is a good eater, sleeps all night in a bed, and when he does wake he'll just play with his toys and his brother until we get up.

All I can say is I hope other fathers who may be in the same situation as myself will read this and find that everything turns out great.

When parents like these first learn that they have a child with Down's syndrome it is of course difficult to come to terms with the diagnosis. Along with the hurt and bewilderment, they have to begin the process of constructing an understanding of what the effect of this means for the child, themselves and the family. The early stages are not a time for making long-term decisions, but a time for parents to get to know their child and to come to terms with the limitations imposed by the handicap. Professionals *should* be there to help in this process, but knowledge, understanding, and sensitivity are needed.

Dave and Mary, both in their mid-20s, had been married for five years and had one son, Simon, who was 18 months old, when they decided another baby would complete their family. Mary was lucky and became pregnant almost immediately. She felt fine throughout the pregnancy and went into labour at the expected time, the delivery was quite normal, and the whole process could be described as a 'text book pregnancy', culminating in the birth of a girl, which she had hoped for – Sarah's name had already been chosen. However, Mary soon became anxious.

Something seemed to be wrong, I could sense it in the attitude of the staff. I was looking forward to giving my baby her first feed, but Sarah was not brought to me. When I asked why I could not feed my baby I was told she was in an incubator, apparently with respiration difficulties. After two days I was allowed to breastfeed Sarah; although she did not suck much my worst fears were alleviated, she was a funny looking little thing, but then most new born babies are so why should ours be different, besides if there was something wrong someone would have told us, wouldn't they?

Four days later Sarah was feeding properly and we were allowed to go home. It was then that I looked at Sarah's card from the hospital, it held all the usual information, date and time of birth, name and weight, then it said – 'Good Down's syndrome' what a funny expression I thought, but it said 'good' so there could be no problem. Three days later the health visitor called and I queried the card, she looked blank and embarrassed and suggested that we spoke to our family doctor.

We made an appointment to see our doctor the next evening, I was a little apprehensive but certainly not ready for the bottom to drop out of my world. Our doctor told us that Down's syndrome meant Sarah had 47 chromosomes whereas other babies had only 46 chromosomes in 23 pairs, this meant nothing to us, so the doctor explained – 'It's a bit like making a cake, you put the ingredients in for an ordinary cake, but accidentally a little coconut falls in, it's still nice, but it has a little extra.' Well that can't be too bad we said, and then the thunderbolt – 'Your child is severely mentally handicapped, a mongol' – I still hate that word, I think it's the ugliest word in the English language, thank goodness it's not used so much these days. We both cried our eyes out, this couldn't be happening to us, what could we tell relatives, friends and neighbours? I felt I'd produced faulty goods, I felt ashamed and as if it was all my fault. Many times I asked WHY ME?

Mary and Dave began to cope; Mary's mother was very supportive. Simon was too young to understand – all he knew was that he had a little baby sister whom he loved, even if she did have funny eyes! However, they had still not told relatives and friends, and Mary found she could not go outside the house because she felt she could not face the neighbours. It was Mary's mother who forced the issue:

One day mum came round and said we could not put off going out any longer, we all needed fresh air. I must admit I put the biggest bonnet I could find on Sarah and covered as much of her as I could with blankets. I felt none of the pride a new mum should feel when taking her baby out for the first time. When I saw a neighbour crossing the road to greet us with a smile on her face I felt physically sick. She pulled back the blankets to look at Sarah, I could see her frowning, but couldn't bring myself to admit that anything was wrong. I tried to act normally but returned home feeling exhausted.

Mary and Dave both loved Sarah but didn't know how to cope or where to go for help. Their regular health visitor was unsympathetic; the only help she offered was to suggest that Sarah be placed in residential care where she could be cared for by professionals. But then a relief health visitor called.

An angel in disguise, that's the only way I can describe her, I can honestly say if this lady had not arrived I think I would have gone mad, I just couldn't come to terms with things. She explained that she had been specially trained to work with handicapped children and their families.

She called three days running. The first day she called I was having a bad day, what I called one of my 'sob days'. She was so sympathetic she just sat and listened, I felt as though a great weight had been lifted. The next day she said I had got to come to terms with Sarah. Once I had faced up to my problems I could begin to overcome them. She started by making me say the word 'mongol', if I could just say it once a barrier might be broken. After bitter crying I said it for the first time, it's an awful word, I never use it, but she explained it was one I was going to hear for the rest of Sarah's life. She also gave me a contact who had a Down's baby. It took me three weeks to pluck up the courage to phone her, and after a long phone conversation we agreed to meet for coffee. It was wonderful to know that I wasn't the only person in the world with a Down's baby and we have been friends ever since, sharing each other's problems and happiness.

Mary was much happier knowing she had someone who understood her problems, and was slowly beginning to accept Sarah as her 'daughter' and not her 'handicapped baby'. She realized that her needs were the same as any other child's, and her biggest need was the company of other children. How could Sarah lead a 'normal' life if she had no normal model? Mary spoke to several mothers in the neighbourhood and arranged a group of four mothers and their toddlers to meet in her house once a week. Instead of helping, this only depressed Mary further. She began to worry about Sarah's floppy limbs and the fact that she was making no attempt to crawl, while other children her age were beginning to walk.

The playgroup that Simon attended suggested that she took Sarah along to see if this would help to stimulate her. Sarah enjoyed the playgroup, and Mary found it more acceptable as the other children were older so she was not constantly comparing Sarah's progress with theirs.

When Sarah was nearly 4 years old the social worker suggested she might benefit from a few hours a week at the local Special School, and an appointment was booked with the paediatrician to assess Sarah's physical abilities:

The assessment went well, there was some concern that Sarah was not yet pulling herself up or crawling, but she was absolutely the hottest thing on a bottom! An appointment was made for us to visit the school . . . When Dave and I arrived at the school my heart was thumping and my stomach churning, how could I think of leaving my little bundle of 'india rubber' with strangers, I hadn't left her since we came home from the hospital. But the school seemed cosy and welcoming and the Nursery teacher did all she could to alleviate any fears we had. Sarah started off attending school just two half days a week and after a few teething troubles we've never looked back.

Sarah is now a well-adjusted 14-year-old, well integrated into the community, attending the local youth club and Gateway club.[1] She is also a member of the Guide company in her area. Mary is fortunate that her child is now well-adjusted, which can be attributed to her constant hard work through Sarah's formative years, but her difficulties could have been greatly reduced at the outset by good professional help with an understanding of the problems she would be facing and by appropriate counselling from the time of Sarah's birth.

Apportioning the 'blame' – feelings of guilt

Parents may begin by trying to attach blame, may feel guilty, may wonder what they have done. This theme of 'parental guilt' is ancient, and has haunted parents through the ages. Each age looks to its own system, culture and practices and asks where have they been violated. In pre-Augustinian times God was blamed, the Middle Ages held association with witchcraft responsible, and the eighteenth and nineteenth centuries blamed immoderate living.

Our present age is no different in this respect: we too look for somewhere to affix blame. Perhaps 'heredity' is the *bête noire* of this age. No matter how carefully it is explained that Down's syndrome is not a hereditary condition, parents still search their own and each other's family background for evidence of mental disturbance. 'Wasn't your uncle a bit . . .?' or some variation of this question, is a regular feature of early counselling sessions. The counsellor can only keep reassuring parents that *they* are in no way at fault. This may be the time to point out that the cause is 'biological' but not hereditary; that it can and indeed does happen to people from all

1. A nationwide federation of clubs for developing leisure activities for mentally handicapped children, originated by Mencap. Information can be obtained from Mencap (address on p. 189).

walks of life, occupations, cultures. It may not be appropriate at this juncture to offer the complicated information about non-disjunction of chromosomes to some parents; to others it would be entirely appropriate. It may well be asked if there is any causal factor or connection with oral contraceptives. Here the answer is less clear. However, as it is a major issue and one which causes much concern, it is worthwhile examining the question in some detail.

The contraceptive pill – possible effects

From a number of researchers working in different parts of the world, Denmark, France, the USA and Britain, have come reports of an increased incidence of Down's syndrome in young mothers along with a slightly decreased incidence in older mothers. However, it must be pointed out that while the 20–34 year-old age group is responsible for the largest proportion of Down's syndrome births in any one year (64 per cent of notified births of children with Down's syndrome in the period 1971–80), again it should be remembered that this is the age group which is responsible for the largest number of births of any kind. This does not explain the *increase* in births of children with Down's syndrome to younger mothers, an increase which appears to have been developing steadily over the past three decades. The most likely cause of the increase is the influence of some environmental factors, and the increased use of oral contraceptives has been suggested as that influence. *There is, however, no experimental evidence to support this suggestion.*

Since such a considerable number of women are now using oral contraceptives it is important to establish what effect, if any, they have on the incidence of Down's syndrome. The following is an attempt to outline the work which has been undertaken on this aspect in order that some of the difficulties of establishing such a connection might be better understood.

Although it has *not* been established that oral contraceptives affect the incidence of Down's syndrome, it is important to consider the degree and possible mechanism of the effect they may have. Studies which have concentrated on investigating the existence of such an effect fall into two categories: studies of babies who have been miscarried and live-birth studies.

Studies of miscarriages

The possibility that the use of oral contraceptives may increase the risk of chromosomal abnormalities was first reported in 1967 when a researcher (Carr) reported a high incidence of such abnormalities in the miscarriages of women who had recently ceased using oral contraceptives. No cases of *trisomy* (i.e. Down's syndrome) were recorded. The bulk of abnormalities were *triploidy* (a non-viable condition where *every* chromosome is in threes instead of in pairs). Carr continued his research over the next few years. He compared 54 miscarriages from women who had ceased using the pill with a control group of miscarriages from non-pill-users. Chromosome abnormalities were shown to be more frequent in the pill group – 48 per cent as opposed to 22 per cent in the control group. The increase was in polyploidy (triploidy and tetraploidy which would be non-viable) with very few trisomy, in spite of the fact that trisomy is the most common form of live birth anomaly. It is worth noting that three out of five miscarriages which had been conceived in a period of between eight and twelve months after discontinuing the pill were in fact trisomic, though no conclusions can be drawn from this as the numbers involved were so small. In 1976, Alberman and her colleagues found a 20 per cent increase in abnormal miscarriages from those who had been taking the pill for longer than eighteen months. This seemed to support the earlier findings of Carr.

A problem which arises in all studies of miscarriages is that of karyotyping – the microscopic examination and counting of chromosomes. For instance, in Alberman's study only 992 out of 2,620 miscarriages were successfully karyotyped. Obviously her numbers were large enough to be considered carefully, but nevertheless they still only reflect a karyotyping success rate of 38 per cent.

Live birth studies

A number of studies have circumvented the problems of karyotyping miscarriages by karyotyping individuals after live births.

A study conducted in 1976 compared the results from two groups of mothers who had used oral contraceptives. One group of 103 who had children with Down's syndrome were matched on age, race, date of delivery and area of residence with 103 control mothers. The results from both groups were very similar. Only one small difference emerged from this study. It seemed that mothers of children with Down's syndrome had greater difficulty in conceiving. The mean interval between discontinuing the pill and conception was two months longer in this group (6.2 months), than the control group (4.1 months).

Lejeune and a colleague in Paris compared the oral contraceptive history of 730 mothers of children with Down's syndrome with that of 1,035 mothers of infants with other abnormalities. These results showed an excess of pill-taking in the 30–38 year-old mothers of children with Down's syndrome. The study, however, was not statistically convincing, since there was a low response rate to the questionnaire from the controls (40 per cent) which may have resulted in skewing of the data.

A further study carried out in 1980 investigated 104 women who had babies following oral contraceptive failure. The malformations from this group were compared with nearly 17,000 other births, but there were no significant differences between the groups of Down's syndrome births; only one Down's syndrome birth resulting from the 104 contraceptive failures. Harlap and Eldor, who conducted this study, combined their results with eight other studies of 'breakthrough' pregnancies. They found eight major malformations in 541 births, which they say is 'similar to the expected frequency in any unselected population'.

To recapitulate – there are no conclusive results from research findings which can *positively* link the use of the contraceptive pill with the birth of children with Down's syndrome. However, a hormonal imbalance has been linked with the causes of Down's syndrome since the turn of the century, and it has been suggested that the hormone balance can be temporarily disturbed after pill use. A return to ovulation may not indicate that normal activity has been resumed.

Read considered the theoretical aspects of the effect of the contraceptive pill on Down's syndrome birth incidences and conducted a small survey himself. He points out that no significant results have been forthcoming from any of the experimental work carried out so far, and concludes that there remains only the *suggestion* of an association.

One study attempted to link young mothers of children with Down's syndrome (not necessarily pill-users) with older women, by suggesting an acceleration ageing process in the former group. However, methodological weaknesses must be pointed out in this study. The criterion for assessing the ageing was the presence or absence of grey hair. A further weakness was that the study was retrospective – mothers were interviewed from between one and eight years after the birth. The findings that grey hair was more frequent among the mothers of children with Down's syndrome can hardly be considered significant in view of the additional amount of emotional stress that the birth and subsequent care of a handicapped child can cause.

Family counselling

The following story of the life and development of a child with Down's syndrome was told by an experienced psychologist who is also an ordained priest.

Jane was born after a normal pregnancy and labour. A few hours after the birth, the doctor confirmed that she was a child with Down's syndrome. She took her first steps at 18 months and said her first words at 2 years. At 2½ she started to attend an 'opportunity playgroup' and at 3½ was enrolled at a day school for children with severe learning difficulties. Here she was placed on an intensive language remediation programme, so that by the age of 7 not only was she talking fluently but she also had a reading age of 6 years. She could count up to twenty and could add numbers up to ten, using counters. The psychologist and the medical officer consulted with both the headmistress and with her parents, and it was decided that Jane should be given the opportunity of integration into the ordinary school. She was therefore found a place in a slow learner unit for children with moderate learning difficulties attached to such a school. Again, Jane progressed well. She required considerable help and support from her teacher but made steady if

slow educational progress. She became much more socially confident than perhaps she would have been had she remained in her
special school.

At the age of 11, Jane had a reading age of 8 years and was
transferred to another slow learner unit attached to her local secondary school. Towards the end of her school career she began to
experience some difficulties. Though she could cope with a limited
range of social activities, her peers had begun to outstrip her socially
and educationally and to have vocational aims which she would
not be able to realize. However, in her last year in school she was
able to attend a bridging course arranged for mentally handicapped
children at a College of Further Education. The career guidance
officer decided that she would fit in well in a sheltered workshop,
and a place was found for her. Jane now lives at home and attends
the adult training centre where she is considered to be one of the
more socially competent members of her group.

Dr Victor Shields went on to say how content her parents were
and how proud and satisfied they felt with her progress. He added,
though, that he wished every child with Down's syndrome could
master skills and adjust so well to social situations as did Jane. Not
all children with Down's syndrome are so fortunate and all stories
do not end on the same note of 'happily ever after'. It is distressing
for parents of a good number of children with Down's syndrome
to be constantly hearing of near normal development and of high
individual achievements when their own child is not making anything like that kind of progress. We do need to recognize the wide
range of ability and rate of development in those children and be
prepared to acknowledge those children who are developmentally
slower and give even more support to their parents. Perhaps if we
could do this we might learn something about our attitudes to all
children. It is so easy to admire the intellectually gifted.

Most admire and cherish a normally developing child. However, many people have mixed feelings when they first encounter a
handicapped child. They may feel shock, repulsion even, helplessness, sorrow and perhaps anger, although such emotions may
not be admitted. All of us tend to fear what is abnormal and
uncontrollable in our lives. Sometimes we may feel enraged that
such problems should even exist. Meanwhile it is important to

realize how families tend to react when they have a handicapped child, and to appreciate some of the stresses on the relationships between family members. Every family, regardless of social class, which has a handicapped child will experience a variety of normal family tensions in addition to the particular stresses of bringing up a handicapped child.

Helping parents and parents helping themselves

Real problems can develop if the whole family becomes disorganized because of the existence, care and management of a child with Down's syndrome. This can arise out of engaging in over-intensive developmental programmes which are extremely time-consuming, in an effort to accelerate development of the handicapped child. Certainly it will do the child with Down's syndrome no good at all if family life does become disorganized and falls apart. It is important that no member of the family feels neglected, particularly other children in the family. Otherwise they will resent the child with Down's syndrome and feel guilty about their resentment. They have a right to normal family life. The family needs to be well enough organized (and for this they may need help from outside the family) to be able to live part of their lives not entirely devoted to the child with Down's syndrome. Interest and time need to be found for other children and for the parents themselves.

It is difficult for professionals not to take over, to tell the parents what to do and what not to do. If they are not 'advising' or 'directing', many professionals feel that they are not fulfilling their professional role. Parents may disagree with the professional and sometimes they may be right! Parents do tend to know best about the daily management of their child and the professional needs to ensure that his or her advice takes this into account. A parent should always insist that when advice is given it is given in a language they understand. Professionals are fond of jargon and anyway it is an easy means of communication among themselves, but advice or instruction or information needs to be clear and understood if it is going to be effective. I was told by a parent recently that '. . . he is operating at the twenty-fifth percentile, er . . . is that good?' And on another occasion, 'I have been told her expressive language is not equal to her receptive language. Is that serious?' (Actually these terms simply mean in the first instance that 75 per cent of the population in the child's age group are making better progress and in the second instance that expressive language, which is the expression of language in speech, is less developed than receptive language, which is the understanding of spoken language.)

Rights and benefits

If benefits are available they should be claimed with no feelings of guilt. Parents of children with Down's syndrome pay their taxes and have every right to any benefits; National Insurance is still *insurance*. Children with Down's syndrome have rights under the law like anyone else, and it is important that they and their parents enjoy these rights and for others to see that they do so.

No family can be defined simply in terms of having a child with Down's syndrome. Whether or not they are good parents, or good people for that matter, cannot be allied to Down's syndrome. It is whether or not the family is able to live a good life that counts, in spite of the handicap.

CHAPTER 11

EDUCATION

When medicine has done all it can, education is the only therapy.

Historically speaking, it is not so very long ago that it was thought that very little at all could be done for the mentally retarded beyond care and protection. The idea that such children could be educated must have seemed like the fantasy of a few idealists whose feet were not really on the ground. In 1838 when Esquirol published the second of his medical dictionaries, *Des Maladies Mentales*, he wrote:

> It is useless to combat idiocy. In order to establish intellectual activity, it would be necessary to change the conformations of the organs which are beyond reach of all modifications.

Thus, the medical model was firmly established. It was a pretty depressing model at that. The message was clear; the impairments causing mental deficiency were believed to be so fundamental that it was regarded as a total waste of time and resources to attempt to change them. By all means it was right to be benevolent, to be kinder in social treatment and perhaps even to move towards the improvement of conditions of custodial care, but any attempts at treatment must be doomed to failure.

It was against this background that Édouard Séguin one year later, in 1839, opened what must be regarded as the first school in the history of special education. It is interesting to note that at this time Séguin was what we would now call an educationalist, having temporarily abandoned his medical studies. It was many years later, in 1861, that he finally completed his medical studies, taking an MD in America. In the field of the education of the mentally handicapped no one would deny the link between education and medicine, yet even today there are those who sit blindly in opposite camps, each refusing to acknowledge the contribution of the other.

The school which Séguin opened was highly successful and astounded many of his former critics, even though it was housed in a hospital for incurables. Séguin was remarkably forward-looking and saw in the early days of his school that the medical model and the hospital setting were inappropriate for purposes of education. He saw the problems arising out of incidental learning by imitation, which today is a powerful argument against segregated schools. Séguin was not easily satisfied. Referring to the many testimonials to his success and to the interest which was now beginning to be shown in his work, he complained that however pleased the Commission which had been set up to evaluate his experiment and the results he had produced was, '. . . they cannot make a hospital into a school, they cannot prevent the contact with epileptics from depraving the idiots, they cannot give me the wherewithal for instruction and all the necessary freedom of action'. Séguin went on to argue that any worthwhile results had been obtained under the most unfavourable conditions, and that he was not able to develop his ideas and methods in his present circumstances. But if such methods had already been shown to work, 'what may I not expect from the hope I have been given of applying the method wider under more advantageous conditions?'

What they had seen must have impressed the Commission, because when they reported back to the Minister of the Interior, Séguin was given a school and also an assistant. The Commission had observed that a physical education programme (perhaps primitive by today's standards but revolutionary at the time) had improved physical fitness, which consequently had advantageous effects on the children's coordination. Their movements were more precise and directed. To many of his poor 'idiots' Séguin had taught reading, writing and simple number skills. Drawing was also an important part of his curriculum. The Commission were amazed that he had been able to introduce his 'pupils' to the concepts of form, size, weight, colour, density, etc. and even to the more abstract ideas of 'authority, obedience and duty', the latter qualities being particularly highly thought of by the ruling classes in nineteenth-century Europe. Altogether, they concluded, he had made his charges 'wiser and more robust'.

It could easily be imagined, from our present perspective, that the pupils Séguin was teaching were somehow of a higher order than those we know as severely mentally handicapped today and therefore would have been more susceptible to educational manipulation and change. This was not so. A report from a visitor from America, sent to observe Séguin and his work, described the pitiful state of the young people sent to Séguin's school. These pupils were also from a wide age range; early intervention had not been invented; indeed, intervention of any kind was refreshingly new:

... many of whom rejected every article of clothing, others of whom, unable to stand erect, crouched themselves in corners and gave signs of life only by piteous howls, others in whom the faculty of speech had never been developed, and many, whose voracious and indiscriminate gluttony satisfied itself with whatever they could lay their hands on.

Such was the state of the candidates for Séguin's school. A similar sight would not be unusual in some of the larger mental institutions in our modern-day civilized societies. Yet the same observer was able to report on the progress of these people after exposure to Séguin's educational treatment:

... properly clad, standing erect, walking, speaking, eating in an orderly manner at a common table, working quietly as carpenters and farmers, gaining by their own labours, the means of existence, storing their awakening intelligence by reading one to another; exercising toward their teachers and among themselves, the generous feeling of man's nature, and singing in unison songs of thanksgiving.

'Awakening intelligence.' It is indeed interesting that this observer, writing in the year 1847, could recognize something which a good many of our present-day psychologists and teachers cannot. With our sights fixed so firmly on measurement by psychometric tests, we tend to forget that it is useless measuring that 'intelligence' which has not been 'awakened' and attibuting to the subject of the test a low degree of 'intelligence', a poor 'mental age' and then setting our sights accordingly. This is expectation fulfilment at its worst. Séguin's expectations knew no limits. And this, it must be emphasized, was with the most pitiful, the most deprived, the most unpromising section of the normal curve of distribution of people with mental handicap.

It became more and more obvious that the old medical model had been hopelessly wrong. Unfortunately, it was only obvious to those with access to Séguin and his now growing number of disciples. It did not necessarily follow that medicine had nothing to contribute, it was simply that pessimistic prognoses had been made, following attempts to change the constitution of people who were mentally handicapped and to seek for a complete cure. Indeed, Séguin owed a great deal to his early scientific training and to his background as a medical student. He saw the retarded individual in the same way as he would see a medical case, where diagnosis came first and then a prescription followed, but for Séguin the prescription was in terms of educational treatment. His first principle was to change the environmental conditions; attending to suitable clothing, food, hygiene, etc. and then arranging for what Séguin described as 'contact with the out-of-doors'. Next came a full and comprehensive medical examination which ignored the mental state but concentrated on the physical and physiological state. Only then did he turn his attention to the educational treatment, beginning with motor control and disorders of coordinated movement. He developed the technique which we now call 'fading' and 'prompting'. For example, on the task of climbing a ladder (a strategy used by Séguin), the teacher would climb some rungs of the ladder from the opposite side, holding the child's fingers against the rungs and encouraging him to release his foothold on the rung. With many trials, each one becomes less dependent on the teacher who holds less firmly, giving fewer instructions, until the child is able to complete the task himself. Séguin also designed many pieces of apparatus for fine motor control, visual perception and matching, geometric shapes to be fitted into matching spaces, for example.

Séguin must also have been the first to employ music therapy to encourage the development of speech. This approach was likely to have been most successful with his pupils with Down's syndrome, for reasons which will be made clear later. The object was simply to intone vowels to music rather than speech, along with training in articulation.

Music was used in other ways too. An English visitor remarked on the relative grace of the dancing of these children whose dancing was accompanied by simple but appropriate music. He also remarked on the singing, saying that '. . . the words were distinctly pronounced, the melody was sung with some force, but not over-loud, the time was well kept, the pause between each verse was distinct, and as far as I could judge, the time appeared correct. In short, the whole piece was executed in a style quite equal, if not superior, to what we are in the habit of observing in the junior singing classes in Great Britain.'

This report is in sharp contrast to one made in Great Britain more than 100 years later. Of course, the subjects of this 1946 report were residents in a mental institution and had received no teaching, encouragement or stimulation. For purposes of this report they were simply expected to 'respond' to music with little or no previous experience and certainly no idea of what was expected of them. Naturally, the conclusions were that people with Down's syndrome (on whom the experiment was conducted) had no sense of time, rhythm or interest in musical activities.

Séguin was well aware that mere training (although that is what he called his approach) was not enough. Simply responding to instruction or reacting to stimuli did not fully equate with learning. He was consequently cautious about aspects of what we know now as 'behaviour modification'. He was critical in this respect of his former tutor, Jean-Marc Itard, commenting that Itard had no par-ticular strategy for developing intelligence. He pointed out that it was easy up to a point to 'oblige the senses to perceive a motion', even to respond to a signal, but he recognized that while the senses are susceptible to environmental control, 'we do not know how to oblige reasoning to function'. He was particularly concerned here with what he described as moral education. By this he did not necessarily mean religious knowledge or even polite and civilized interactions, he meant knowledge of an act; to have an idea of meaning, to have some foresight into the possible consequences of an act.

All visitors to Séguin's school came away extremely impressed by the change and progress which were taking place among the pupils. One such visitor referred to an individual case in a report made in 1847:

This being, who in 1843 had been in so strange and apparently hopeless condition, could now read, write, sing and calculate. I had already noticed him in several manifestations of attachment and other moral qualities. I now saw him happily engaged, making good use of implements with which, if placed in his hands a few years ago, he would doubtless have inflicted serious injury.

This visitor goes on to describe all kinds of activities taking place, shoemaking, carpentry, handicrafts, agriculture and all under minimum supervision and carried out with a 'normal' degree of skill. He also echoes in his report what had been expressed by others:

As no notice had been given of my intention to inspect the institution, I have every reason to believe that what I witnessed was nothing more than the ordinary daily routine.

It was Séguin's work with the mentally handicapped that influenced Maria Montessori, the first Italian female to graduate in medicine. After successfully applying Séguin's methods to the education of handicapped children in Italy, Montessori recognized that the same approach could be applied to the education of non-handicapped infants. She attempted this with great success, and eventually Montessori schools could be found in many parts of the world where normal, bright children were being taught by methods originating from Séguin's contribution to the education of the mentally handicapped.

How far have we progressed since that time, or have we in some aspects taken a few steps backward?

Early intervention

Séguin had clearly and dramatically demonstrated that intervention at any age could bring about profound changes in behaviour, skills and the quality of life for the mentally handicapped. However, it is obvious that the earlier intervention takes place, as long as the goals are appropriate to the age and stage of development of the child, the better it will be for him. Time is not wasted which could be better used, and developed skills, particularly those concerned with self-help, make life easier and more pleasant for those around the handicapped child. Basically, all the arguments which can be presented to demonstrate the value of nursery education for 'normal' children apply equally, if not more so, to the handicapped. It is doubtful that early intervention will raise the limits of the eventual ceiling of possible achievement, but it will certainly make it a more pleasant journey getting there, and for all concerned. That is, of course, unless too much pressure and effort are put into this early education. Too much pressure can make learning a misery for the child, can cause over-anxiety in the parents, and can lead to neglect of others in the family. Cunningham's Manchester studies have shown that there might be some immediate gain related to the degree of intensity applied to intervention activities but there appears to be no long-term gain. Nor does it make a great deal of difference *when* such intervention begins. Infants who are started on programmes later tend to catch up quickly with those who started earlier. The level of attainment will always, of course, be related to the intellectual capacity of the child, along with other social and emotional variables.

A phenomenon which is frequently misleading in an assessment of the effectiveness of early intervention programmes is that of reducing hidden deprivation. For example, if after a programme of early intervention has begun (or coincidental with its beginning), the child has some improvement in health, or the need for spectacles is recognized, then this disadvantage is removed and there could be an upsurge of development, regardless of the new programme; but of course the child will be better able to benefit from the programme as well. Also, there may have been very low expectation on the part of the parents, and when these expectations rise, the results of intervention tend to rise with them. This is certainly what had happened with Séguin's extremely deprived subjects before he began to work with them.

Apart from frequency and intensity, according to Dr Cunningham, it does not seem to matter which professional is involved with the family, providing the professional is properly trained and is well aware of the objectives. It might be a psychologist, it might be a health visitor or peripatetic teacher (i.e. one who is not attached to a school, but travels around where needed). Where many professionals are involved there is a need for communication and cooperation. Working individually there is always the danger of conflicting advice which, apart from confusing the parents, can lead to inter-professional wrangling instead of interdisciplinary cooperation.

On the whole it seems better that intervention with professional guidance is carried out in the home rather than a clinic. The surroundings are familiar and less threatening and the apparatus is chosen from objects within the home, the child's own toys for example. Of course this can result in isolation and it is probably best if advantages can be taken of both worlds, with regular but not too frequent visits to a clinic or centre. This will give the mother an opportunity to meet other mothers and to compare notes. The child might, with luck, be attending a nursery school which will provide an opportunity to mix with other children.

School years

Special schools or special schooling was the outcome of Séguin's work. He had devised the educational treatment on the basis of instinct, observation and scientific principles and was reinforced and encouraged by its success. When one examines the fundamental principles, aims and objectives which Séguin developed it can be seen that they are not so very different today. Perhaps they have been adapted to meet the needs of a handicapped child growing up in today's world, and maybe the names of the techniques have changed as they have been refined, but by and large they have not changed much. This, more than anything, demonstrates the vision of Séguin. Of course one advantage we have today is the capacity and techniques to evaluate the effectiveness of any programme or process. It is a great pity that we do not take advantage of *these* kinds of approaches. Often enough we are all too ready to be satisfied that everything is all right if it looks right. If something appears to work it might be for other reasons than from a particular form of intervention.

The object of much present-day research into learning behaviour of children with Down's syndrome is to make our teaching more effective by giving a deeper understanding of the learning processes in these children. Some research is concerned with questioning the myths which have grown up around Down's syndrome and some is concerned with improved ways of measuring success, both in the children and in our investigation. Altogether there is a tremendous amount of effort being made by research workers in order for us to reach a better understanding of ways and means to meet the developmental needs of people with Down's syndrome.

It is amazing that a short time ago, no more than about thirty years, it was not generally expected that a child with Down's syndrome would learn to walk or to talk with any degree of normality, let alone learn to read and write. At least, text books of the time spell out a gloomy picture, and new mothers of children with Down's syndrome were told not to expect any real progress or development.

Happily we now seem to be returning to the optimistic days in Bicêtre, France, where Séguin had his school, and where he did the impossible, like teaching reading, writing, calculation, singing, drawing to 'ineducable' children – some of whom were undoubtedly children with Down's syndrome. Séguin does not record it because at the time Down's syndrome had not yet been isolated from other forms of handicap, but it is more than likely, as it is today, that they were among his best scholars.

It is no longer remarkable to find a child with Down's syndrome reading fluently, in fact it is expected. Research studies are examining the best ways to facilitate the skill. Also attempts are being made to discover the best and most effective ways of teaching any skill.

Some interesting work has recently been completed by two Edinburgh researchers, Duffy and Wishart. They have provided evidence which suggests that 'error-free' learning seems to suit these children best. Most children actually need to encounter errors in their school learning. They learn from their mistakes. Not so the majority of children with Down's syndrome; they appear to go for what has been called 'failure avoidance', even to the extent of failing deliberately at a task well within their comprehension, just so that they will not be expected to move to a more difficult task which they are aware they are not able to do. Very small steps, each one meeting with success, are more likely to be profitable.

It is not appropriate to go deep into the complex subject of 'intelligence' here. In order to give a detailed account of differences of rate of growth or development of intelligence in children with

Down's syndrome it would first require a technical explanation of the concept of intelligence, a subject which occupies many volumes in the psychological literature. Readers who would like an up-to-date account of intelligence in Down's syndrome are referred to the work of Dr Janet Carr of St George's Hospital, London. What should be said about intelligence in Down's syndrome is that just as no two children with Down's syndrome are physically identical, the same must also be said of variations in intelligence. In fact, the range of intelligence at each age and stage is probably wider in the Down's syndrome population than in the so-called normal population. This of course has implications for almost any statement which is made about learning and learning behaviour in children with Down's syndrome. With this caution in mind there are certain generalizations which can be assumed, though to repeat, not all children with Down's syndrome will adhere to them. Attention span, for example, is shorter. Not just willingness to pay attention, but more errors tend to be made the longer concentrated attention is required.

Short-term memory is weaker, causing difficulties in retaining information long enough to process it properly. Long-term memory, while appearing to be remarkably good, is in fact also weak. Facts which most of us will discard from our long-term memory, or never allow to be deposited there in the first place, will often be retained by children with Down's syndrome, thereby not leaving space for important things to be remembered. In other words, they are unselective.

There is a tendency for children with Down's syndrome to handle knowledge as being divided into distinct and separate pieces of information without forming links, or, as it is put, 'discrete elements'; they tend to have difficulty in handling more than one dimension at a time, thereby reducing the ability to reason, e.g. $A + A = B$, or $A + B = AB$.

Creativity should form an important part of the curriculum for children with Down's syndrome. The present-day urgency to teach basic skills in literacy and numeracy we can easily result in neglect of aspects of creativity, or their reduction to less important levels. It is noteworthy that Séguin, over 150 years ago, placed music and drawing alongside reading and writing.

Music has always been associated with Down's syndrome, the first reference being made about ten years after the condition had been described by Langdon Down. Then Shuttleworth in 1900 spoke of 'the mongols' great love of music', adding that their 'idea of time as well as tune is remarkable'. Tredgold in 1908 repeated the same description but added 'a marked sense of rhythm'. These musical characteristics have now entered the folklore, and even those with little or no acquaintance with children with Down's syndrome will usually remark: 'They are very musical, aren't they?' Eden was probably nearer the truth when he wrote in 1976 that

there is a popular impression that all mongols are affectionate, exuberant, happy, biddable and musical. It is perhaps safer to say that mongols are individuals like the rest of us and are not obliged to be any of these things.

All these statements regarding 'musical mongols' are conjecture, or impressions based on casual observation. In order to test out this characteristic experimentally, Evonne Ching, a Chinese colleague, and I embarked on a series of experiments in which we measured responses to rhythm and time in children with Down's syndrome, along with control groups of children who were mentally handicapped but did not have Down's syndrome and mental-age-matched non-handicapped children. The results showed that the Down's syndrome group did not have anything like a marked sense of time and rhythm but they were identical in competence (in incompetence too) to the group of 'normal' infants. Both of these groups were, however, significantly better than the other group of mentally handicapped children.

Further work has shown us that children with Down's syndrome are quicker to respond to musical activities, but only when they are well taught. Unlike the results coming from those in mental hospitals and reported in the 1946 studies referred to earlier, our results, coming from a school where careful attention was given to music and movement, were more in accord with those observations made in Séguin's school so long ago. Our observers made identical comments, speaking of 'grace' in the movement to music, of the quality of the graceful dancing. This certainly made us wonder what we have been doing during the past 150 years or so.

Equally important is the value of painting and drawing in the development of children with Down's syndrome. Young non-handicapped children use their drawing as a second language, so to speak. Concepts and dawning realizations of the world around them can be expressed in their drawing, and they can use this medium as a means of coming to terms with their environment. Young children, like mentally handicapped children, have little spoken language with which to express their ideas and no written language. As they grow older and acquire more skills, the delightful representations made by young children are often discarded in favour of imitations of what they perceive as adult art. Children with Down's syndrome are very much later in acquiring language skills and will rarely become so proficient that they will be able to express all they wish to express in sophisticated language. Consequently drawing and painting as a means of wider expression take on so much more importance. All the childlike symbols become more elaborate but the intention to communicate remains the same. Another Chinese colleague, Carmen Au, and I have noticed this in cultures as different as England and Hong Kong.

Generally speaking, though children with Down's syndrome will be slower and perhaps different in their learning, they are a delight to teach. They have certainly earned their reputation as the undergraduates of the defective world.

Which school?

The movement since the publication of the Warnock Report in 1978 has been towards integration for children who are mentally handicapped into 'ordinary' schools. There is a good deal to be said for social integration of children rather than segregating them into special schools for the handicapped. Basically the same principle applies as it did in 1839, when Séguin was appealing for a school separate and away from the mental hospital. Séguin complained that the mentally handicapped were exposed to the influence of the bizarre behaviours of mentally disturbed people. This is particularly unfortunate for children with Down's syndrome because a well-known and undisputed characteristic is their 'skill' as imitators. It would indeed be fortunate if only the best behavioural characteristics were transmitted: if, for example, autistic children could be influenced by the out-going sociability of children with Down's syndrome. But, human nature being what it is, things usually work the other way round – it is all the worst behaviours of any group or individuals which become common.

The other side of the coin, however, needs careful examination. Special education cannot be had cheaply. Teachers need special training to understand the needs and different learning strategies of the handicapped. Extra help will be necessary in classrooms where vast differences in the rate and style of learning occur. We have now in Britain an accumulation of nearly twenty years of experience of special schooling for the severely mentally handicapped. If this is not to be wasted, the organization and concept of integration must be more than simply moving children from one school to another.

The experience of Italy is an example of good intention without sufficient attention to possible consequences.

The Roman professor Paolo Meazzini, a strong advocate of the *principle* of integration, is also an advocate of caution. The problems, he points out, are not confined to Italy. Studies carried out on the effectiveness of integration have drawn attention to a number of major factors which cause poor results:

1. The absence of a sound methodology backing the educational and rehabilitation programme. As a result the quality of staff performance lowers as their expectations drop.
2. Inadequate training of staff so that they are deprived of effective professional skills.
3. Uses and abuses of psychometric testing, which opens the way to a self-fulfilling prophecy. Many writers have pointed out that there is very little hope of educating a child if one believes that nothing or very little can be done to improve his intelligence.
4. Modelling, by means of which inadequate behaviours shown by peers are added to the already low functioning skill repertoire of the handicapped child. Inadequate, or unacceptable behaviours are not confined to special schools.

As to the Italian experience, Meazzini had this to say:

... laws were passed which abolished all special schools and enforced mainstreaming of all handicapped children, irrespective of the type and severity of the handicap. Neither school setting nor school personnel were prepared to meet these new demands. The move towards mainstreaming was thus ideological and emotional with few rational guidelines being provided that could make mainstreaming possible. In addition no experimental programme was set up to find out how to plan and implement mainstreaming. The result of this typically Italian approach can easily be imagined, and has in fact come about: chaos as regards services and frustration on the part of teaching staff. This may well lead to legislative steps that may dramatically limit mainstreaming and restore segregation once again.

We have been warned. Meazzini summarizes by giving top marks to Italian legislative bills and social sensitivity but very low marks to the Italian way of planning and implementing mainstreaming. Unfortunately imagination is not sufficient to solve such a complicated social and educational problem as full integration.

CHAPTER 12

THE NEW TECHNOLOGY

The genesis of the 'new' technology in education belongs to the early 1960s and what was then called 'teaching by machinery'. The psychological concept behind the new approach was not new even then, as it originated with Skinner in the early 1950s. Put simply, the theory works like this: the learner is presented with a stimulus, i.e. something which attracts the attention and provides some information (it is irrelevant how simple or complex the stimulus information). The learner responds to the stimulus. Of course the more evocative the stimulus, the more it demands some response. The learner is presented then with further information (feedback) which gives an indication of how appropriate, or correct, was the response. This procedure can carry on in a continuous chain until a final goal has been reached. The thinking which goes on in the mind of the learner as decisions are made about responses is called by psychologists 'information processing'.

These machines were quite crude and mechanical but caused a good deal of excitement in educational circles because it was demonstrated that the learning of straight facts – even complicated mathematical facts as well as simple word recognition tasks in reading instruction – could be learnt much faster by this method. Some disquiet was expressed concerning the possible effects of isolating children to working with a machine and of losing the stimulating effect of interacting with other children.

By 1965 several large engineering companies were collaborating to bring this approach into their apprentice training programmes. Exciting possibilities were on the horizon for what looked like a revolution in educational practice. None of this, however, was directed to the really slow learner. At this time, it must be remembered, the slow learner was what we would now call 'moderately' handicapped; the severely mentally handicapped had not yet become the responsibility of the education authorities. It is interesting to record that a writer of the time who considered the handicapped as being possible beneficiaries of the new approach continued: 'With mentally handicapped children the role of teaching machines will only be evaluated healthily after sufficient programmes have been devised' (*déjà vu?*). Maybe sufficient programmes were not devised for anyone, because before the end of the decade the teaching machine was quietly put away and forgotten.

In recent years this older concept has returned but with a much more efficient and sophisticated technology. Computer Assisted Learning or CAL has great potential for meeting some of the basic learning needs of mentally handicapped children, if only we organize ourselves well enough to exploit it. Early reports which began to appear in 1980 were anecdotal but encouraging, particularly on teaching simple skills. Comments were made about the capacity of CAL to keep the attention of even severely handicapped individuals.

An enthusiastic advocate for the application of this new technology to the learning behaviour of handicapped children is Dr A. K. Ager, a clinical psychologist working in Birmingham. Commenting on these early reports, he refers back to the old programmed instruction literature and maintains that the work could have benefited from extending its findings. Ager suggests that though the range of applications is broadening to include even the profoundly multiply handicapped, '. . . the work is for the most part still fragmentary, and the progress of research is thus constrained by the lack of an integrated literature'. From a practical point of view there is a further difficulty. Design errors can often result in a programme made to teach a simple skill but requiring a more advanced skill to operate it. Obviously there is a need for collaboration between psychologists, special educators and programme designers. A few have managed this, and the results suggest that such collaboration should continue and spread. Ager describes one such project which gives a good example of what can be achieved. The project was called 'Micromate'.

'Micromate' seems to meet the conditions which teachers and parents of the handicapped would ask. It is cheap and portable and is based on firm scientific understanding of the learning processes in mentally retarded children. While the system was designed for the Sinclair 2X Spectrum, it is now compatible for use with other microcomputers such as BBC, Apple and Electron. An ordinary television screen can be used for the visual display, and the programmes are loaded from a standard audio cassette recorder.

Though the concept keyboard or even the normal microcomputer keyboard might be suitable for some of the more advanced children with Down's syndrome, the designers of this system played safe and, recognizing that many may not have fine motor control, they developed a touch sensitive screen and switch box which can be plugged into the microcomputer to allow such children to operate the programmes. The touch sensitive screen is designed to attach to the television screen so that the operation proceeds when the appropriate part of the panel is touched. This system is also helpful to those children who cannot associate a remote keyboard with images on a screen. The switchbox is available for those who can accommodate this concept but do not have sufficient fine motor control to operate a keyboard. This switchbox consists of a wooden box with three large mushroom-shaped switches mounted on the box.

The programmes are designed for simple concept learning such as colour discrimination and size judgement, and usually involve matching exercises.

The system has been scientifically evaluated through extensive tests with children who are severely mentally handicapped and attending a day school. They worked on a trial and error method, first being taught certain discrimination skills the conventional way and then by the Micromate method. Of course, some learning from the first method might have carried forward, but even allowing for this the results were quite convincing and the rapid development of these children was reported as 'clearly encouraging'.

This approach is consistent with the description of the preference shown by children with Down's syndrome for error-free learning (see page 117).

This system was explored with a child with Down's syndrome by a colleague, Rosemary Fraser, and me, in a home environment.

The mother had no experience of microcomputers – her first encounter with the apparatus was when it arrived along with Rosemary and me at her home. There were no complications as the child was quickly able to handle the keyboard. The procedures were demonstrated to the child and his mother at the same time, though a few extra loading instructions were given to the mother! We then asked her to note how the child used the programmes and how he progressed. One week later the mother was delighted. She said that James was working the computer before breakfast and was 'beating' his two non-handicapped brothers.

Several things were learnt from this practical experiment and from the child's approach to more complex discrimination tasks. First, we had assumed that a good deal of repetition and consolidation at each step would be the best learning procedure, but this was not so. The best procedure turned out to be short periods at each stage, but each stage needed to consist of very small steps to the target. James quickly became bored with a stage after he had mastered the principle, and he needed to be rewarded by his own progress. However, his mother reported that he was aware when the task was approaching his limit and at this point he would stop. This again is consistent with the 'error-free learning' results of Duffy and Wishart.

Apart from evaluations of the Micromate system showing significant improvement in simple discrimination tasks, there are also reported incidental gains in such areas as attention span.

Another group of programmes which are very popular as well as useful for children with Down's syndrome (and their brothers and sisters) are simplified and scaled-down versions of standard computer games. With the ever-decreasing costs of microcomputers they are now within the purchasing possibilities not only of a wide range of mental handicap services and voluntary groups but also of the average family.

The software for the Micromate system is available from:

Toys for the Handicapped
Micromate Software
Stourport
Hereford and Worcester

A touch-sensitive screen overlay system is also used in part of a programme designed for adults. This is a programme designed by Canadian researchers which begins with discrimination activities. The touch sensitive screen again makes it possible to answer questions by pointing to the answers on the screen. Another special feature of this Canadian system, bearing in mind that this CAL was prepared for adults, is that the computer programme will respond to speech so can cater for users who are non-readers. The programmes for this system are the Basic Concept Packages, and the speech system is known as the Rocky Mountain Hardware Supertalker. They report success with adults on banking, buying, budgeting, coin computation and time-telling.

Further information on these systems can be obtained from:

The Vocational and Rehabilitation Research Institute
3304 33rd Street, NW
Calgary
Alberta T2L 2A6
Canada

A review of research in CAL has identified four major research findings:

1. The computer assists learners to reach educational objectives.
2. Learning by computer saves 20–40 per cent of time over normal conventional teaching.
3. Retention is as good as, or superior to conventional teaching methods.
4. The learner's reaction to good CAL is positive.

If the exciting potential of Computer Assisted Learning for children with Down's syndrome is not to be lost, it is necessary to bring together a variety of people with different areas of expertise; this is not an easy task. If software is to be designed which is appropriate to the needs of children with Down's syndrome, the programme designers and experienced teachers should cooperate with interested educational psychologists, all working together to evaluate results. Then the programmes need to be marketed, so the involvement of a publisher is necessary. There is the need and I am sure there is the will, but such a research project would be fairly costly and equally difficult to organize. Perhaps some research group is already busy at work on such a project!

CHAPTER 13

ADOLESCENTS AND ADULTS

There have been many studies concerned with the development of *infants* with Down's syndrome; studies covering their physical, intellectual and social development. As a result, guidance has been offered to parents on a range of strategies for early intervention in the development of skills in these areas.

A good number of studies have been conducted on the growing *school-age child*. These cover the fundamental issues of levels of intelligence, perception and learning. They have also been concerned with the practical application of theoretical concepts to such areas as language development, reading, social skills and more recently to the growing movement towards fuller integration into mainstream schools.

There is, however, a paucity of literature and relatively few experiential investigations into the development, needs and problems of the adolescent with Down's syndrome, and almost none which look into the continued development into adult life.

This situation is not really surprising since it is not very long ago that the majority of people with Down's syndrome were not expected to reach adulthood, and those who did survive were very often accommodated in mental hospitals where they could be quietly forgotten by all except those who were immediately responsible for their care. Even the wealth of literature and attention to the earlier years, which has been so significant in bringing about improvements in the development of children with Down's syndrome, does not have a long history. Indeed, before the end of the 1960s it would have been difficult to find studies on Down's syndrome outside medical literature.

The upsurge of interest among other professionals such as psychologists, sociologists and educationists came about through the influence of two major forces: first, the parents who organized themselves into pressure groups to make their needs and the needs of their children more widely known, and second, an Act of Parliament which was passed in 1971 bringing all children, regardless of the degree of their handicap, under the care and jurisdiction of the Ministry of Education (now the Department of Education and Science). This removed them from the jurisdiction of the Ministry of Health (now the Department of Health and Social Security), who were till that time responsible for their care and protection. Parents had earlier fought the battle to have the designation and description 'ineducable' changed to 'unsuitable for education in schools', though changing a classification does not always bring about changes in practice.

There are at last healthy signs that similar initiatives are being taken in respect of adolescents with Down's syndrome. A few excellent studies have been produced on these adolescents over the last four or five years One such study, published very recently, is unique in the scientific literature. Sue Buckley and Ben Sacks have presented the results of their investigations in attractive book form in a language that is accessible to parents; it actually loses nothing in detail and accuracy for the professionals either! The results are properly tabulated and the evidence presented as clearly as (possibly more clearly than) in any scholarly journal. The book is privately published and all proceeds go towards research into the needs of adults with Down's syndrome. Full details of how to purchase this book are given in the section on further reading (p. 187).

One question that must always be asked of any researchers publishing their findings is: can the study be replicated for contrast, confirmation or support? This study by Buckley and Sacks meets all the criteria for scientific quality. One very interesting departure from the time-honoured method is the way they have humanized the study by describing details of the daily life of some of their 'subjects'. Of course, in fairness to the publishers and editors of scientific journals, it must be said that space would not permit them to publish studies at such length.

In this discussion on adolescents with Down's syndrome it is worth examining some aspects of the lives of the real adolescents from the book. The adolescents represent a wide range of ability. This is an important feature, as has been pointed out before; it is no service to parents to paint a glowing picture of outstanding progress by the exceptional person with Down's syndrome and to ignore the majority who make steady but unremarkable progress. It would be as unrealistic to expect all adolescents with Down's syndrome to have a driving licence, a well-used typewriter, an entertaining clarinet and facility in a couple of languages (there are adolescents with Down's syndrome who have achieved these things) as it would be to expect all young people to achieve first class honours degrees at university.

Some highlights from the biographies of four of the adolescents have been extracted for comment. One is above average in intelligence and one below, the other two are average boys with Down's syndrome.

Alan

Alan is 15 years old and is the youngest in his family. He has a sister and two brothers. Both his parents are employed. Alan is a little precocious for a youth of his age with Down's syndrome: 'He is beginning to show an interest in the opposite sex and enjoys kissing girls at discos.' His parents are not over-concerned about his apparent sexual development, even though they reported him as coming home from school after lessons on sex education and enlightening them about the facts of life! His conversation sometimes centres around getting married and having children. This gives some worry to his mother, who is not sure how to deal with this and either puts it off or laughs it off. Alan has a great sense of fun and enjoys imitating people. A rather sad aspect of his story is exemplified by an incident when he shaved off his eyebrows because he said they made him look handicapped. In fact he had the same style of eyebrows as the rest of his family. Unusually for a youth with Down's syndrome, he was aware of his handicap, his difference from others; not surprisingly, this difference distressed him.

Alan belongs to the top end of the ability range of people with Down's syndrome. It can be seen, however, from this small part of Alan's adolescent life that being relatively able also brings its problems. There is a further interesting issue raised here, one that naturally concerns many parents, possibly Alan's parents too, though their strategy for dealing with the concern is to *say* they are not over-anxious. This is the problem of sexual development.

Parents of boys may be less anxious than parents of girls about this aspect of growing up, but it is still a matter for concern even in terms of the boy's acceptance among young people of his own age, and the reaction of other parents to his attention to girls. What the neighbours think is a powerful influence on our lives, whether we wish to admit it or not. Unfortunately, apocryphal tales are told of an uncontrollable maniacal sex drive being a principal character-istic of the Down's syndrome male, usually when a community home or hostel is proposed in a 'respectable' neighbourhood. Such tales could not be further from the truth. As far as is known, there is no recorded case of a male with Down's syndrome becoming the father of a child. There is also no evidence of males with Down's syndrome initiating overt sexual activity with females. They display affection, certainly, but they never cause problems which might be feared by the mothers of young females. As Smith and Berg have put it, '. . . in general, individuals with the syndrome can hardly be ranked amongst those who may be said to constitute a sexual hazard to others. If some caution is indicated, it will most likely be required in the context of the Down's syndrome individual possibly being sinned against rather than sinning.'

Perhaps in the interests of accuracy one doubtful case should be mentioned, where it was reported that a child had been fathered by a 'mosaic' male with Down's syndrome (see Appendix, page 167, for full description of mosaicism), but this could hardly be described as typical, as the proportion of normal cells could have been quite high.

Real heterosexual desire seems to be low, and a good deal of 'interest in the opposite sex' is imitative play, learnt behaviour and a desire to be seen doing what others do. Often, of course, real, honest, simple displays of affection can be misunderstood. The following describes a not untypical incident:

A teacher was taking a group of handicapped young people round a supermarket as part of their social skills training. At the check-out, one 15-year-old youth with Down's syndrome noticed the pleasant attractive girl at the till, so without the slightest inhibition he went round and gave her a hug, much to her surprise and alarm. The teacher was able to explain, and happily the girl was even flattered. There was nothing wrong with the behaviour itself – it was simply acted out in the wrong place under the wrong circumstances. This is an important lesson, which is difficult for teenagers with Down's syndrome to appreciate; they must learn that 'good' behaviour means also according to time, place and occasion. If *real* integration into the community is to come about, then these lessons are more important than many others.

There is a natural tendency to treat adolescent boys and girls with Down's syndrome as though they were little children. Unreasonably, we then wonder why they have great difficulty in learning grown-up behaviour. This was noticeable at a recent international conference where a young man with Down's syndrome was present. Despite the fact that he was behaving in a quiet, dignified and adult way, a number of people – among them professionals – patted his arms or ruffled his hair as they would a 3- or 4-year-old, or they ignored his presence if they were about to indulge in 'serious' conversation. We must ourselves learn to behave appropriately towards people with Down's syndrome before we start demanding appropriate behaviour from them.

Returning to Alan and his dawning sexuality, there is every reason to believe he will cope in spite of experiencing some problems; he is bright.

Mary

Mary is at the other end of the scale. She is 17 and the youngest of three children. She did not speak at all until she was 8 years old, and even now only uses sentences or phrases of three or four words. Her speech is such that she cannot be understood by strangers. Mary's parents speak regretfully about the neglect they feel they have given to the other children in order to cope with Mary and her needs. Now they also recognize that they have been equally neglectful of their own social needs. They do not want to think about the future, about what Mary will do when they can no longer care for her. Their future is only considered in the very short term; they hope that she will be able to go to a training centre when she leaves school. Mary has an imaginary friend and spends most of her time in the 'company' of this friend, often blaming the friend for any of her own wrongdoings.

This 17-year-old girl seems to be quite content with her own company and is oblivious to the problems her presence is creating around her. This is a typical picture of a 'retarded' adolescent with Down's syndrome. There is a catalogue of everyday things which Mary cannot do: tell the time; know the days of the week; describe the weather; describe anything about herself except her name.

This case highlights the need for a family life which is not completely centred around the specific needs of the handicapped child. These parents have devoted themselves almost exclusively to catering for a severely handicapped child, and on their own admission have sacrificed the needs of other members of the family to this end. They regret not having had proper advice in the girl's early years. It is in cases like this that the well-trained professional is invaluable. One can only imagine what might have been had there been some good family support. More than likely the household was pretty glum during Mary's early years, as they counted the things she was unable to do and waited hopefully for signs of better things to come. Then came the gradual and further disappointments when those hoped-for attainments were not achieved. It is also likely that they were expecting too much, expecting Mary to do things that were quite beyond her capabilities. This is just as bad as expecting too little; the long-term lower expectations tend to follow when expectations have been initially too high. It is more difficult to adjust downwards than the other way round. Delight follows when the 'hidden deprivation' of low expectations is enriched by appropriate intervention and small but significant achievements are recognized.

Mary's imaginary friend is her strategy for coping with a situation which is out of her control. She *can* control her 'friend', who remains at the same level as herself. Many, more able, adolescents with Down's syndrome relax by this strategy, often projecting the friend on to some favourite doll. Conversations can be rehearsed for hours in this way and are non-threatening. It is a stage which many 'normal' children go through in the early years, and which they leave when confidence in reality is established.

Mary would probably never have made significant achievements, but the family might have been a great deal happier if her disability had not so dominated it. However, it is still not too late to improve matters for this family. Mary eats well and tidily and can help herself to food and drink with the minimum of assistance. She is quiet and usually well-behaved. The parents can now take her out with them and enjoy meals in restaurants without stress and anxiety.

Kevin

Kevin is 16 and has two younger brothers. He has good table manners and needs no assistance with his food. He can even make himself simple meals of sandwiches or toast and prepare a hot drink. Kevin knows how to use the cooker grill and will do so without supervision. His speech is the problem. He uses three or four words at a time but is difficult to understand, which causes some frustration; at times he will cease talking altogether. Kevin has no problems finding amusements for himself: he likes pop music and sings along with his favourites, he enjoys television and his own company.

Alternative forms of communication might be offered to Kevin. Drawing, as well as being another form of communication, might reduce his frustrations. A good speech therapist might be able to help. Perhaps some training in sign language could supplement Kevin's articulation problems. This must only be developed as a supplement to speech, because elaborate sign language is only useful if other people can read it. It is not wise to rely too heavily on sign language, despite the help it can give. It does, however, seem to ease the tension and frustration so that speech becomes more possible with relaxation.

Kevin has brought a great deal of joy and happiness to his parents, in spite of his demands on their time and energy. Perhaps the other children have not had as much of their parents' attention as they and their parents would have liked, but this has been more than compensated for by the growth in tolerance, patience and understanding in the development of his younger brothers. Kevin's parents have higher hopes for the future and look forward to some kind of work for Kevin which will be interesting for him. Perhaps later he could become more independent by living in a small hostel with minimum supervision.

This is a summary of part of an optimistic story of an *average* teenage boy with Down's syndrome. His parents have high expectations but at the same time are realistic when considering his likely achievements. As far as employment goes, even in times of high unemployment, as David Lane has pointed out, there is no reason why the handicapped should bear the brunt of it. Kevin is a lively, capable boy and it has been demonstrated over and over again that such boys can hold down certain jobs, making good employees. Such jobs need not be routine and uninteresting; for example, assisting in parks and gardens can be enjoyable employment. People with Down's syndrome often have the patience to preserve some of the old crafts which are fast disappearing; once taught a skill they are as competent as anyone. The hotel and catering industry is always short of labour, and people with Down's syndrome make loyal and conscientious workers. The Down's Syndrome Association employs a girl with Down's syndrome as its office junior.

The hostel idea is also gaining favour with the Social Services. This is a far better solution than passing away time in a large mental hospital. Initial problems encountered by placement in accommodation of this kind have usually been caused by attempts to re-accommodate people who have spent too long in mental hospitals and become institutionalized. The sudden change has been too much for them. The use of hostel-type accommodation has been very successful in Scandinavia. Given this kind of environment from the start, with proper preparation and well-trained, well-motivated staff, the continuing process of development for the handicapped adult is much more likely to succeed.

Sharon

Sharon is 16, with an older brother and a younger sister. She is even more accomplished than Kevin in cooking, being able to cook a variety of fried foods and also use the oven for some dishes. She can read simple books and does so for enjoyment, though her educational skills are varied. She cannot, for instance, read or write a simple message or her address, though she knows her address and will say it. She cannot tell the time, though she can count and compute simple sums. This does not extend to a real understanding of money values, even though she can recognize the different coins. Sharon seems to enjoy the normal pursuits of a teenage girl – pop music, television, swimming and dancing.

Though at the moment Sharon is showing no particular interest in boys, her parents are worried about the future and the problems which might arise.

This teenage girl is quite self-sufficient within a limited capacity and has the means to live a decent and dignified life. Obviously she will always require some help and supervision, however minimal. There is one serious problem, however, certainly as far as her parents are concerned, and that is: how can she be protected from sexual exploitation? Will she become pregnant if given too much freedom? This is felt to be a much more serious problem for Sharon's parents than it is for Alan's.

Let us examine the purely biological problems of possible pregnancy. First let it be said that up to ten years ago Smith and Berg recorded only 23 cases of pregnancy in females with Down's syndrome from all the medical literature from all parts of the world. Others *may* have occurred since and there *may* be some pregnancies which have not been recorded. However, it is worth bearing in mind that in the civilized world such pregnancies would be regarded as highly unusual and the births would take place in hospitals, thereby making a record almost inevitable. These births have occurred out of a population of perhaps somewhere in the region of 6 or 7 million. The chances of pregnancy then do not appear to be very high. Though menstruation appears to be reasonably normal, a very large proportion of females with Down's syndrome show no ovulation; the suggestion is therefore that females with Down's syndrome have very low fertility levels.

Reports on those pregnancies which have been recorded are as would have been expected. Theoretically, half the offspring would have been Down's syndrome and the other half would not. There would also be the expectation of a higher than average rate of spontaneous abortions in such pregnancies. Of the 24 full-term babies recorded by Smith and Berg, 9 had Down's syndrome, 2 were mentally retarded, 10 were normal and 3 were stillborn (see Table 5).

Table 5. Babies born to females with Down's syndrome [adapted from Smith and Berg (1976)].

Description of child	Age of DS mother at birth of her child
Normal female	25
DS male	30
DS female	19
Retarded male	30
Retarded female	29
Normal male	—
Normal male	22
DS male	23
DS female	21
Stillborn male twins	14
Normal male	21
Stillborn female	20
DS male	22
Normal female	18
Normal female	27
DS female	18
DS male	17
Normal female	19
Normal female	30
Normal male	16
DS female	23
Normal female	25
DS male	20

The chances of a pregnancy occurring in Down's syndrome are so extremely low that there should be no great cause for alarm in this respect. A moment's thought should make it clear that sterilization, apart from being an ethically unacceptable violation, is also unnecessary. Sterilization can only prevent a highly unlikely pregnancy anyway. It cannot prevent sexual violation. Sterilization cannot prevent rape or incest – indeed it might even encourage it; neither can sterilization prevent sexually transmitted diseases. There can be no substitute for a high level of care and protection by parents or by staff charged with the care of people with Down's syndrome, or indeed any other handicapped person. This is the only kind of approach which will ensure that opportunities for promiscuous behaviour are not so abundant.

When I recently asked a now retired director of a residential community for handicapped people how many pregnancies there had been in the community during his thirty years as director, he thought for a few moments and then answered: 'I would guess about two a year, on average.' He then thought again and added, 'I am speaking now about the community staff, is that what you wanted to know?' He had no hesitation when I told him that my inquiry was about the handicapped residents; he said, 'Oh, you mean the handicapped; none!'

It would be difficult to elaborate on all the findings from the fascinating study on adolescence by Buckley and Sacks, as they consider almost every aspect of teenage life, but they do conclude that the main implication of their survey is that 'parents need positive support and accurate information from the outset.' The children need good health care and expert education throughout their childhood. Among many, perhaps the most important statement they make is that 'Most young people with Down's syndrome are able to achieve far more than most professionals still realize.'

An important aspect of two other studies which were addressed to the development of adolescents with Down's syndrome is that they are longitudinal. In other words, the same group of children have been monitored throughout their growing years.

Janet Carr followed up 54 children with Down's syndrome for twenty-one years. She reported on their progress at 4, 11, 16 and 21 years, and her descriptions of the changes in these families and children make interesting reading, especially as she compared their progress with a group of non-handicapped children born at the same time. A similar kind of study was also carried out by Shepperdson in South Wales. Ann Gath did a large scale single study of 94 boys and 99 girls covering the age range of 6–17 years. Gath focused particularly on the families and the emotional and social concerns of the families, while Carr's study was aimed particularly at the children and their development. Naturally, though, something of both sides comes into each of these studies.

Later years

There can be no doubt that people with Down's syndrome are living longer. This must be a result of better living conditions, better health care and, hopefully, an increasingly healthier attitude to handicapped people. As far as meeting the needs of adults with

Down's syndrome, we have hardly yet begun to scratch the surface. But their pressing needs are beginning to be recognized. We have not yet begun to address the development and concerns in the later years.

The effects of Alzheimer's disease continue to cause problems in a general deterioration of functioning after the age of 40 (the onset might be much earlier), and since there have been suggestions that this disease seems to be present in every person with Down's syndrome after that age, a good deal of research is going into this problem. Alzheimer's disease, the disease of ageing, claims far more people than those with Down's syndrome, but Down's syndrome is particularly interesting to those researching into this problem. One reason is because there is in Down's syndrome such a large population known to suffer from the disease, and another is that the symptoms of Alzheimer's do not seem to be so severe in Down's syndrome. So, while the most grudging interpretation of the interest from the point of view of Down's syndrome might be that they make 'good' subjects for the study of the disease, people with Down's syndrome will certainly benefit from any successful results of such research.

A great deal of effort, imagination, time and cost has gone into providing the best means for the development of children with Down's syndrome, from birth until the end of the school years. If this is not to be wasted, we need to turn our attention and imagination more seriously towards the further development of the late adolescent and the adult.

Theoretically it is possible for a young person with Down's syndrome to remain in full-time education until the age of 19; however, there are regional variations in availability of educational places for young people between the ages of 16 and 19. A number of Colleges of Further Education run life skills and other courses, but much will depend on the availability of such a course within travelling distance from a person's home. Sheltered Workshops and Adult Training Centres provide some places, but the kind of training and the kind of work available may not always be the most appropriate to the needs and the ability of the young adult with Down's syndrome.

An opportunity was lost in 1971 at the time of transfer of responsibility from 'Health' to 'Education'. Junior Training Centres became Special Schools and were then obliged to employ qualified teachers. Surely this was the time for Adult Training Centres to become the equivalent of Special (Secondary) Schools. But legislation was as always, inflexible, and could find no way out of the restrictions imposed by a chronologically determined school-leaving age. Many teachers would agree that by the time the average child attending a special school for severely handicapped children (formerly known as E S N(s)) had reached the age of 16 years, they had in effect come to the end of their 'primary' school education. Why turn them out of school on account of their age? It would have been a bold move to have brought 'education' into the Adult Training Centres.

Barbara Furneaux makes the obvious point that 'maturation continues after the age of 16, so the severely subnormal can benefit from further training and education'. She goes on to say that the task of educating the handicapped is inevitably a lengthy one, extending beyond the teens and into the twenties because of the slow rate of development. The recommendation that training centres should become the responsibility of the education authorities and not the Social Services was made in Section 10 of the Warnock Report. The Warnock Committee were referring to separate education facilities within the centres; the overall responsibility for general and continuing development might well remain the responsibility of the Social Services.

It might be asked what the Adult Training Centres are training adults for? Very few trainees indeed leave to go into open employment. The manager of one centre, talking to David Lane, was confident that many of the trainees with Down's syndrome were capable of keeping a job. With more than twenty years' experience in this type of work, the manager thought that adults with Down's syndrome were grossly underrated. He went on to say that there has been a tendency to develop them into 'trained handicapped persons'. In other words, trained to become handicapped. Lane sees ATCs as places which provide day care for the mentally handicapped. Perhaps it is now time to campaign for the development of services for the adult with Down's syndrome towards real education and training, so that the potential which was stimulated by early intervention can somehow approach realization.

CHAPTER 14

HELP FOR THOSE WITH DOWN'S SYNDROME

The professionals

It would be unreasonable to expect all professionals to have an intimate knowledge and understanding of the needs of children with Down's syndrome and their parents. The condition of Down's syndrome may have occupied only a very small part of their professional training. Only recently has it taken on a higher level of importance in professional education, as more has become known about the condition and of possibilities for effective professional intervention. A good deal remains to be done in in-service training of those professionals who have not had the opportunity to up-date their knowledge. Perhaps even more difficult is the need for inter-disciplinary cooperation between the different professionals involved. Conflict between professionals can result in creating a worse state of affairs than if they had not been trying to help in the first place. To this difficulty must be added the real suspicions which exist between parents and professionals.

Happily, more and more professionals are beginning to take a specialist interest in the mentally handicapped and in Down's syndrome in particular, but there is still a long way to go before the Warnock principle of parents as partners becomes a reality.

Before turning to the problems of encounters with professionals and the kinds of problems involved, it is necessary to make clear what kind of professional involvement might be expected. This can only be a general survey, also not all services described may be available or be similar in all authorities, though if it is considered essential there are ways of enlisting the particular professional skill required. These services will apply mainly to the pre-school child, though many continue well into the school years and sometimes beyond.

The midwife

The midwife provides the first line of care for the mother and baby. Her role is to help to create a strong bond between the mother and her baby and to monitor their health. She is responsible for visiting the mother and baby at home up to the tenth day or, if necessary, up to the twenty-eighth day after birth.

The health visitor

The health visitor has a duty to visit a mother and child within the first ten days and then to visit the home regularly until the child begins schooling. These visits should allow her to form a close relationship with the family, to observe the development of the child within the family and to give general help and support.

The specialist health visitor

The specialist health visitor is a recently created post where the health visitor has a particular interest, or specialist training, in physically and mentally handicapped children. Apart from the role of health visitor as described above, she should also be able to offer practical advice on bringing up a handicapped child and to liaise with other Health Service staff and other agencies, in order to provide a comprehensive service.

The idea of specialist health visits came originally from the Warnock Report, which had recommended a 'named person' to enable professional support to be given to parents with greater speed and with less formality. Leicestershire were quick off the mark by providing two such specialists within a year of the Warnock Report being published. Little by little the appointment of specialist health visitors began to spread throughout the country, sometimes as a result of organized parental pressure as it became clear to them the help that such a visitor could be. Referrals to this specialist are made by health visitors, district nurses and sometimes directly by the parents themselves.

The general practitioner

The general practitioner's role is to provide continual care for the child and the family and to provide any primary health care which the child or family may require. Of course when a child with an obvious genetic handicap like Down's syndrome is born in hospital the GP is not immediately involved, but he or she should always be put fully in the picture immediately, at least before the mother and her child are discharged from the hospital. The GP may refer the child to:

(i)   The health visitor.
(ii) Other community nursing facilities.
(iii) Specialist services in mental handicap, which would include expert help as required from a psychologist, physiotherapist, occupational therapist, speech therapist or social worker.
(iv) A consultant in paediatrics, who may refer the child for further assessment to a specialist clinic, or unit.

The paediatrician

The paediatrician assesses the health of the child at regular intervals and is able to refer to any specialist professional help that may be necessary, surgical, ophthalmic, orthopaedic or any other.

The physiotherapist

The physiotherapist is the person who is concerned with helping to improve the child's bodily coordination, muscle tone, and motor control, for example in sitting up straight, or in learning to walk.

The occupational therapist

The occupational therapist is concerned with teaching children individual skills such as feeding, washing, dressing and general

Even when parents express anxieties and suspicions about their child's development, these are too often disregarded by professionals ... Many parents need to be in contact with someone who can see that their anxieties are taken seriously and followed up. .

Mittler and Mittler, writing in 1982, felt that this need introduced by Warnock must lead to a 'consumer model' approach where the starting point is the individual family. Partnership, they said, involves '... a full sharing of knowledge, skills and experience in helping children ... to develop as individuals'. Mittler had observed earlier, in 1979, that there were obstacles to partnership: lack of experience with professionals, lack of confidence, negative experiences. All these can lead to intolerance on the part of parents. Also memories may be faulty; feelings of guilt may be inappropriately off-loaded on to the nearest convenient person. But perhaps it is for the professionals, who almost invariably maintain greater detachment from the situation, to communicate to the parents their desire for both parties to work together. It is the degree of success which is achieved that determines the way parents will perceive the relationship.

A former student of mine, Liz Hanson, interviewed a number of parents in 1985, asking them about their experience with professionals. From the verbatim reports of her interviews there seem to be good grounds for optimism, though those professionals who had been difficult or less than useful came in for a good deal of criticism, most of it being divided between educational psychologists and social workers. Hanson observed, however, that when parents reflected on their past experiences with professionals, memories of encounters which had annoyed, depressed or saddened them were the ones that they recalled with the greatest ease. Satisfactory relationships were dealt with shortly with phrases such as, 'We've no complaint about ...' '... was all right'. She also reports that parents were generous in their praise of professionals who they felt had responded to them as individuals and had respected their views.

Sometimes it was the organization that was at fault as much as the professionals. Mrs Campbell was nearly collapsing under the strain of sleepless nights and frequent hospital appointments. She often had to attend different departments of the same hospital, but as there was no central coordination of appointments she experienced repeated journeys and long waits with a fretful child. Many of the assessments seemed to Mrs Campbell to be unnecessary, and no one explained to her why they were being carried out. Far from being regarded as a partner, Mrs Campbell felt that she was tolerated but was unimportant.

Some of the comments from parents in the Hanson survey are revealing:

Mrs Adams: All along we feel we've had the so-called experts tell us, who live with him, what he can and can't do.

Mrs Bell: The doctor turned round and said, 'Peter's never going to be able to look after himself, he can't even feed and dress himself', which was a load of rubbish. We tried to explain that Peter was very nervous in front of him, he couldn't do anything. But he wouldn't listen.

Mr Docherty: We didn't properly have the opportunity to have our point of view heard. I mean we *told* them, but they thought we weren't worth listening to. I mean I *know* my own kid's capabilities, I *live* with him . . . they must think I'm bloody stupid.

Mrs Bell acknowledged when things went well and gave credit to the professionals who had helped:

We had a marvellous social worker at the time; but for her we'd never have got as far as we did.

And another:

Mrs Ellis: This particular social worker, she was marvellous, she allowed us to make decisions as parents and then go back and say what we'd chosen.

Teachers in special schools were highly praised by the parents, even by those who thought their children had been wrongly placed. Parents were very quick to recognize commitment:

I mean, we've always found his teachers to be very positive and super people, doing all they can and delighted with the progress he's making.

They've turned John from a no-hoper at 10 into . . . he can read, he can write . . . we can't thank them enough.

The school she's in is very good, the headmaster's brilliant. Quite often we go up, we never ring them up, we just go. We say, 'Let's go and see how she's going on', and we're always made welcome.

There are many examples of parents' comments reported in this study, but all of them testify to the positive outcomes to encounters with professionals which were warm and friendly and where they felt that a real dialogue had taken place. If there is no trust or common ground between the parent and the professional no treatment, however sound, is likely to be successful. Parents need to have faith and confidence in those prescribing the treatment. The following story is all too typical of what is *believed*; whether true or not, there can be little success until barriers are broken down:

We didn't see a lot of the psychologist, probably because we didn't agree with her ideas. In the end we asked to change and we went to another psychologist, who . . . even then . . . I mean he was very nice and everything but I think he's been briefed, obviously, by the last psychologist. We didn't get on any better, so, well, what can you do?

We have still a long way to go in training our professionals to be better communicators and to work together as inter-disciplinary teams. When parents become equal partners in such teams, the all-round development of our handicapped children could be much improved.

Voluntary associations

There are a good number of voluntary associations concerned with mentally handicapped children and their families, ranging from the Royal Society for Mentally Handicapped Children and Adults to the small societies which care specifically for the needs of minority handicaps such as the Turner's Syndrome Society. Other organizations have pioneered education for handicapped children, as for example the Rudolph Steiner Trust, and yet others have devoted themselves to making homes for handicapped people such as Home Farm Trust. However, it is the Down's Syndrome Association which is concerned exclusively with those people with Down's syndrome and their families. This organization is a good example of parent professional cooperation. Of course, a good many of the professionals associated with the Down's Syndrome Association are parents of children with Down's syndrome as well as being professionals. It is sometimes forgotten that there is no law of immunity which prevents professionals from also being parents.

One such parent was Rex Brinkworth, who was head of the Remedial Department of a large secondary school in Birmingham in 1966, when his daughter was born with Down's syndrome. In view of his profession he had always taken an interest in under-achieving children, but now as the parent of a child with Down's syndrome his interest focused not just on his own child but on others with the same condition and on the needs of their parents. In 1970, together with a group of parents and professionals in Birmingham, he formed the Down's Babies Association. In those early days of parent organization it was subtitled 'Help for mongol children'.

In 1976 it changed its name to the Down's Children's Association, and with its headquarters at the Quinbourne Centre in Birmingham soon began to spawn branches in all parts of the country. The first regional branch had already been formed in 1973, covering London and the South-East. In 1981, with the cooperation of Birmingham Polytechnic where Rex Brinkworth was then a lecturer, the Associa-tion created the National Centre for Down's Syndrome with Rex Brinkworth as its director. By 1983 the central office moved to London with the appointment of Maggie Emslie, a former speech therapist, as its first full-time executive director. Another change of name followed. Realizing that children with Down's syndrome grow up and still need support and care, the Association became the Down's Syndrome Association. The head office, under its second director, Sue Brooks, is at 12–13 Clapham Common South-side, London SW4 7A A, and has a staff of six with five voluntary professional advisers.

The Down's Syndrome Association has described itself as having a mission. That mission is to create and develop a climate that will enable people with Down's syndrome to realize their full potential as people with prospects.

The Association helps by encouraging parents and professionals to bring out the best in people with Down's syndrome. Self-help groups have been set up so that parents and local professionals in health, education and social services can share their experience and help each other to adopt a positive approach to solving problems. Information is provided by a team of experts to anyone who seeks it about education, health, teenage problems and life after school. Additionally, the Association promotes research into ways of improving life across the whole age range of people with Down's syndrome. Underpinning all its activities is the London-based Resource Centre, which holds a wide range of specialist publications and practical learning aids, toys and audio-visual material. The centre, situated within the head office, is also an important meeting place for people with Down's syndrome, their families, professionals and friends of the Association. Among other things which the Association does is provide a counselling service for parents at times of shock and distress. It also aims to create greater public awareness of the potential of people with Down's syndrome and a more sympathetic understanding of their needs, together with a greater respect for their right to lead fulfilling and useful lives. The Association firmly holds the belief that Down's syndrome in a newborn baby is not a justification for it being allowed to die.

Rex Brinkworth, now retired from his full-time job at Birmingham Polytechnic but remaining as Honorary Director of the National Centre, sums up his own attitude:

Experience has led me to form the conclusion that the child with Down's syndrome has always been handicapped as much by the ill-chosen title 'mongol' with all the assumptions and prejudices the word provokes, as by the condition itself. A great deal of retardation takes place after birth and is to a material degree avoidable.

We aim to provide the means of eliminating this avoidable element in their retardation as far as possible, and to offer a measure of justice to this much misused and misunderstood group of human beings who differ from ourselves not so much in kind as in development.

Developments overseas

A remarkably quiet but important revolution is taking place in many parts of the world. Quite apart from huge organizations like the Down's Syndrome Congress of the USA and the large state organizations in Australia, there are others which tell a story of a less threatening world than we see daily on our television screens.

I have been privileged to join together with Catholics and Protestants in Northern Ireland as they work together towards the development of their children with Down's syndrome. In India a Down's Syndrome Association was formed two years ago, with a committee consisting of Sikhs and Hindus under the guidance of Professor I. C. Verma, Professor of Paediatrics at Delhi. In Mexico Professor Sylvia Escamilla, a dynamic parent and educationist, founded a special school for children with Down's syndrome, the 'Instituto John Langdon Down'. Sylvia Escamilla recently managed an astounding coup by bringing together all the Latin American countries and becoming the first President of a Latin American Down's Syndrome Association. In Zimbabwe the Down's Syndrome Association involves both black and white, taking into consideration only the needs of their children and their support for each other. Hong Kong recently formed its Down's Association with Chinese and English, Australian and Japanese parents. Jonathan Chamberlain, an English father of a baby with Down's syndrome, and Carmen Au, a Chinese teacher in a special school, have worked together to establish their young and vigorous Association. Carmen has now been appointed as Hong Kong's first fulltime executive director. Between them, they produce a professional style magazine, DS News. This newsletter is half in English, from the beginning to the middle, and half in Chinese beginning at the back. I have attended a reception given by the parents and people with Down's syndrome in Prague, where an Association flourishes. Dr Rene Eminyan, an obstetrician and also the parent of a girl with Down's syndrome, has with his associates who run the Down's Syndrome Association on the island of Malta just opened a new Centre in Valletta. Carlo Piccenna, a parent and retired naval officer, has mobilized Sicily and directs the Centro Piccolini Down in Catania. Dr Georgio Albertini, a paediatric neurologist, runs the largest assessment and treatment centre for children with Down's syndrome in Italy from his clinic at the Ospedale Bambino Gesù in Rome. Dr Albertini is not a parent of a child with Down's syndrome but is a professional who has tremendous devotion to children with the condition. New efforts are being made to help children with Down's syndrome in Tanzania with the work and help of the Rev. Philip Kutta, a Catholic priest. Under the guidance of Professor

Jean Rondal, Professor of Psychology at Liège, a new European Down's Syndrome Association has been founded. The Spanish Downs Association, with the help of Professor Flores and his wife, continues to grow. The list could go on. John Langdon Down has given his name not only to a single pathological condition causing mental handicap, but to a worldwide community of people with potential.

APPENDIX: THE BIOLOGICAL BASIS OF DOWN'S SYNDROME[1]

In this section we will endeavour to explain some of the biology that we need to understand in order to learn a little more about Down's syndrome. Clearly this is not meant as a medical text, but as an introduction for the interested reader. There are three sections:

1. Background Biology
2. Cell Division and Human Reproduction
3. How Does Down's Syndrome Occur?

If the reader has a basic biological grounding, and is familiar with the cellular nature of tissues, mitosis, gametogenesis and meiosis, he or she may prefer to start reading at Section 3.

1. BACKGROUND BIOLOGY

Cells

Human tissues, like other living tissues, are made up of microscopically small cells (see Figure 3). These cells can be of many different shapes and serve many different functions. They may be stuck together (e.g. in skin), suspended in a fluid (e.g. blood), or even surrounded by hard deposits (e.g. bone). However, cells do have many things in common. One common feature is that the majority of cells divide, so that tissues may grow or be repaired. Sometimes cell division may form special new cells, such as eggs or sperm. Another common feature is that all human cells (except red

1. This appendix chapter was written in association with Jonathan Steele, BSc., M.Ed.

blood cells) contain an area that may be stained dark. This area is called the nucleus (see Figure 3). The nucleus is the 'control centre' of the cell and it is within this nucleus, especially during cell division, that we must look in order to understand more about the biology of Down's syndrome.

Inside the nucleus

As early as the middle of the nineteenth century scientists noticed thread-like structures inside the nucleus of the cell. However, it took over 100 years, until 1956, to establish exactly how many of these threadlike structures, or *chromosomes*, were contained in the nucleus of a human cell. Of course it is now well established that there are normally 46 chromosomes inside the nucleus of each human cell, and at certain times during cell division they may be observed microscopically and at these times can be photographed. The photographs may be then cut up, sorted, and the chromosomes arranged into pairs, each member of a pair appearing almost identical, or *homologous* (see Figure 4). Depending on when they are photographed, the chromosomes may either be seen as single threads or as a double thread joined together at a certain point (the centomere) to form a rough X shape. Each ⟩ of the X shape is known as a *chromatid*. Scientists have assigned numbers to each of these pairs, so that individual pairs may be identified. The chromosomes are therefore numbered 1 to 22, plus one pair of sex chromosomes (either XX in a female or XY in a male) to make 23 pairs in all.

It is on the chromosomes that all our biological information is carried – from the shape of our big toe to the colour of our hair – and a lot more vital biological and biochemical information as well. All this information is carried inside every nucleus of every cell in the body.

However, in the nuclei of people with Down's syndrome there is an extra number 21 chromosome, making three rather than just the normal two chromosome 21s. But what is it that happens to cause this extra chromosome to appear? To enable us to understand this better we need to know a little more about how cells divide, how eggs and sperm are formed and what happens at the moment of conception.

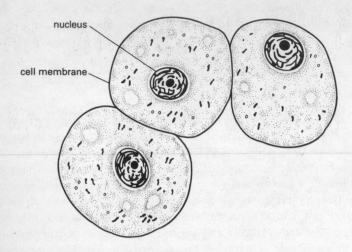

nucleus

cell membrane

Figure 3. Some animal cells.

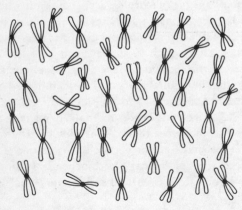

Figure 4(a). Human chromosomes as they appear scattered under the microscope.

2. CELL DIVISION AND HUMAN REPRODUCTION

What happens to the chromosomes when a cell divides? Before cell division the chromosomes make a copy of themselves so that they appear as a double thread (see Figure 4). Every individual chromo-

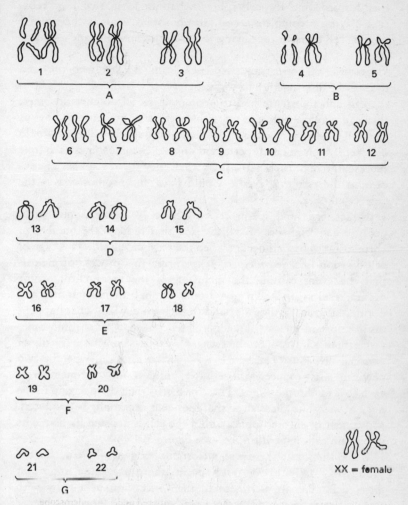

Figure 4(b). Human chromosomes arranged in standard format.

some then splits in half longitudinally, one thread (or *chromatid*) from each chromosome moving to one end of the cell, the other moving to the opposite end of the cell. Two new nuclei are therefore formed, and the cell splits in half to form two new cells, each having a complete set of chromosomes. This is the normal type of cell division, occurring in most human cells, and is called *mitosis*.

However, at conception two special cells, the egg (or *ovum*) and the sperm, fuse together to form the *zygote* (fertilized egg). If both the egg and the sperm had the complete set of 46 chromosomes, then the zygote would end up with twice as many chromosomes as normal! Clearly it would not function or grow properly, and would die. Yet if both egg and sperm had only 23 chromosomes each (one representative of each pair), then when they fused together at conception the resulting zygote would have 46 chromosomes – the correct number.

In fact, eggs and sperm *do* only have 23 chromosomes each, because a special sort of cell division that reduces the number of chromosomes by half occurs when they are produced. This type of cell division is called *meiosis*. It is during this process of meiosis that the event causing the inclusion of the extra chromosome occurs, resulting in Down's syndrome. But first we must understand normal meiosis. Figures 5(a) and (b) help to explain what happens during normal meiosis, but only show one pair of chromosomes rather than all 23. As can be seen, this process consists basically of two cell divisions. The first is a *reduction division,* whereby two new cells are produced whose nuclei contain only one member of each pair of chromosomes. These two cells then divide again in the normal way (like mitosis), so that four cells can finally be produced. Movement of chromosomes within the cell is assisted by filaments of protein called *spindle fibres* (see Figure 5).

While this basic theory of meiosis holds generally true for the production of both eggs and sperm, there are some important differences that are pertinent to the conception of a baby with Down's syndrome, and therefore need explaining. However, before continuing it is important that we have the concept of *mitosis* and *meiosis* clear, so let us summarize them. Mitosis occurs in all cells except when egg or sperm are being produced, and ensures that new cells always have the same number of chromosomes. Meiosis occurs only when eggs or sperm are being made, and ensures that the number of chromosomes are reduced by half.

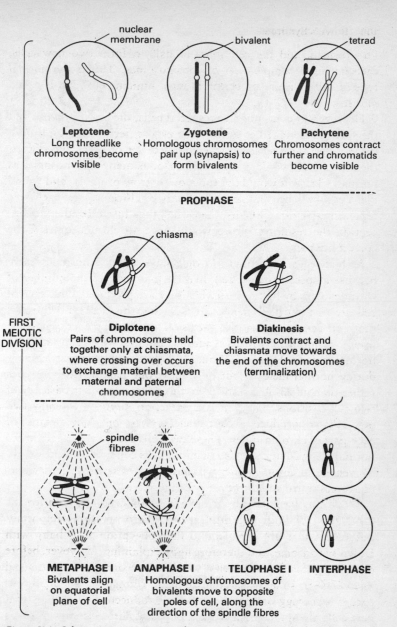

Figure 5(a). Schematic representation of meiotic division showing the behaviour of one pair of homologous chromosomes (or chromosome behaviour during the stages of meiosis).

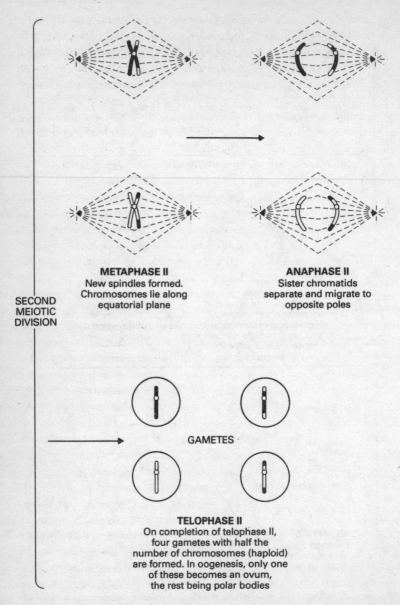

METAPHASE II
New spindles formed.
Chromosomes lie along
equatorial plane

ANAPHASE II
Sister chromatids
separate and migrate to
opposite poles

SECOND
MEIOTIC
DIVISION

GAMETES

TELOPHASE II
On completion of telophase II,
four gametes with half the
number of chromosomes (haploid)
are formed. In oogenesis, only one
of these becomes an ovum,
the rest being polar bodies

Figure 5(a) (continued).

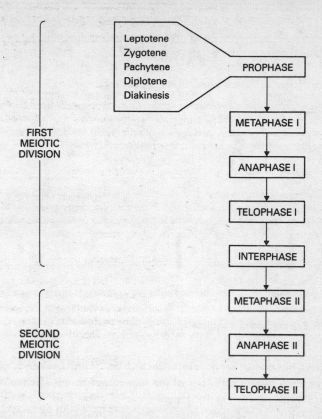

Figure 5(b). A summary of the different stages of meiosis.

Production of eggs

The production of eggs is called *oogenesis*. Surprisingly (and unlike sperm production in men) this process has started before the female child is born. Inside the ovaries, cells called *oocytes* start the process of dividing by meiosis to produce eggs. However, this process becomes held up, or suspended, during the first meiotic division. At this stage all the eggs that the female will ever produce have been

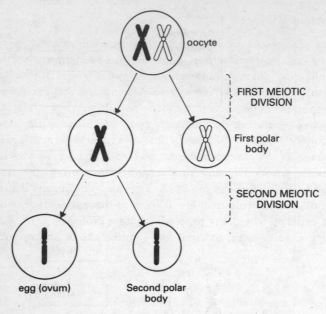

Figure 6. Egg production (oogenesis).

prepared, but no further development will occur until puberty, when one egg each month will 'ripen' (or sometimes more – hence non-identical multiple births) until menopause occurs. This 'suspension' half-way through the development of eggs is probably an important factor in explaining the maternal age effect on Down's syndrome births; the eggs of a woman over the age of 35 have obviously been 'in suspension' for more than fifteen years longer than those of a 20-year-old. Hence these potential eggs, suspended at a fairly vulnerable stage of development, will have had more time to deteriorate in some way. The other important factor in oogenesis is that when an egg-producing cell (or oocyte) undergoes meoisis only *one* egg is produced rather than the four that might be expected. The other cells that are produced are called *polar bodies*; these degenerate and are lost. Figure 6 summarizes oogenesis, leaving out the details of meiosis and showing only one pair of chromosomes for clarity.

Production of sperms

Sperms are formed by a process called *spermatogenesis*. Sperm-forming cells (*spermatocytes*) divide by meiosis to form sperms, but unlike the situation in oogenesis, no polar bodies are formed. Also unlike oogenesis, there are many spermatocytes dividing to make sperms at the same time, so that while the woman usually produces only one egg each month, a single ejaculation from a man may contain 200–300 million sperms. Moreover, spermatogenesis only starts in the male at puberty, and from this period onwards sperms are constantly being produced. Sperms are not, therefore, held up half-way through meiosis as eggs are. This means that the sperm of a 40-year-old man are as fresh as those of a 20-year-old, which explains why many people (including Professor J. M. Berg, see page 5) believe that paternal age is unlikely to be an important

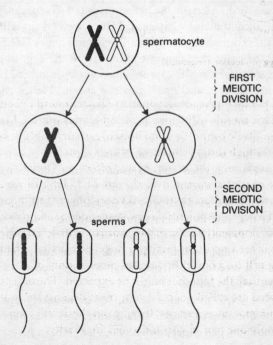

Figure 7. Sperm production (spermatogenesis).

factor in the conception of a baby with Down's syndrome. Spermatogenesis is summarized in Figure 7, leaving out the details of meiosis and showing only a single pair of chromosomes.

3. HOW DOES DOWN'S SYNDROME OCCUR?

Trisomy 21, non-disjunction and Down's syndrome

As has been mentioned, the majority of individuals with Down's syndrome have one extra number 21 chromosome in the nuclei of all their cells. Hence they have three rather than two of these particular chromosomes. This type of Down's syndrome is referred to as *trisomy 21* ('three chromosome 21s'). But how does this happen, and is it anyone's fault?

The error usually occurs during the production of eggs or sperms, when either chromosome pair 21 fails to separate properly during the first meiotic division, or the chromotids fail to separate properly during the second meiotic division. Hence we end up with an egg or sperm that contains two number 21 chromosomes (see Figure 8).

Usually the extra chromosome comes from the egg. In this situation the zygote (fertilized egg) would receive two number 21 chromosomes from the egg, and one from the sperm. Hence the zygote would be trisomic for chromosome 21 (see Figure 9).

About 80 per cent of babies born with Down's syndrome have their extra chromosome because of unsuccessful chromosome separation at the first meiotic division. This process of non-separation of chromosomes is called *non-disjunction*. In actual fact, non-disjunction can also sometimes occur during ordinary cell division (mitosis). While the vast majority of individuals with Down's syndrome have the condition because non-disjunction happened during egg or sperm formation in their parents (and usually during egg formation), non-disjunction during ordinary cell division becomes important in a rare form of Down's syndrome called *mosaicism*, or *mosaic Down's syndrome*.

But before explaining mosaicism, let us squarely and plainly address the question of 'fault'. It is unfortunate that parents, particularly mothers, can experience feelings of guilt on giving birth to a child with Down's syndrome. They harbour an impression that

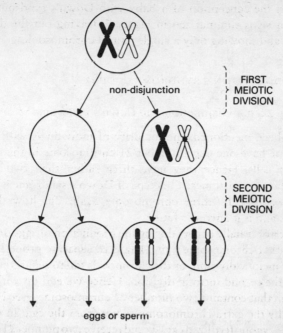

eggs or sperm

Figure 8. Non-disjunction during egg or sperm production. (N.B. Non-disjunction may also occur at the second meiotic division.)

they are in some way at fault, or to blame. It is most important to point out that parental 'fault' does not enter into human genetics. Down's syndrome occurs because of unexpected events happening in the complex processes of cell division. No one can anticipate or avoid such individual spontaneous events, since they are determined by factors quite outside parents' control. Parents may feel guilty, and we sympathize with this, but these feelings arise from the normal emotional reaction to a difficult and traumatic event, and have absolutely no basis in scientific fact.

What is mosaic Down's syndrome?

Stated briefly, mosaic Down's syndrome occurs when only a proportion of the body's cells have got the extra number 21 chromosome (i.e. are trisomic), the others being normal. This is sometimes refer-

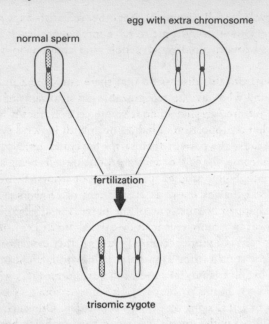

Figure 9. Fertilization of a trisomic zygote.

red to as incomplete Down's syndrome or partial Down's syndrome. However, it is rare, and a number of independent studies have shown that mosaicism seems to be recognizably present in only 2–3 per cent *of the population with Down's syndrome.*

Mosaicism may be suspected if the diagnosis of Down's syndrome is in doubt. This may come about when fewer of the typical physical features of Down's syndrome are present, giving a general impression of the condition, but initial genetic tests have revealed only normal cells. Subsequent tests may find some trisomic cells.

From this we may expect people with mosaic Down's syndrome to have generally higher intelligence levels than those with full trisomy 21. However, it may be unwise to predict intellectual function from genetic findings, as the situation seems unclear. Scientists are divided in their views of intelligence levels in people with mosaic Down's syndrome. Some report intelligence levels of individuals with mosaic Down's syndrome throughout the whole range of expected levels for full trisomy 21. Yet other scientists expect people with mosaic Down's syndrome to have intelligence levels that fall somewhere between unaffected people and those who are fully affected.

It follows from this discussion that there could be a number of people around who have no recognizable physical signs of Down's syndrome, yet are carrying some trisomic cells. In fact it has been suggested that a proportion of babies born with Down's syndrome are born because the parents themselves have undiagnosed mosaic Down's syndrome, the egg- or sperm-producing cells being affected. From dermatoglyphic studies (palm and foot prints) Penrose suggested in 1965 that as many as 10 per cent of Down's syndrome births may happen because one of the parents is affected by mosaicism. However, a more recent study carried out in 1985 suggested that 2.7 per cent is a more accurate figure. Further evidence for this type of effect comes from a number of individual reports where children with full trisomy 21 have been born to mothers who have themselves been found to be carrying some trisomy 21 cells, yet showed no physical signs of Down's syndrome. One such mother had two children with Down's syndrome, the first being born when the mother was only 19. Another mother was 22 years old when she gave birth to the first of her two children with Down's syndrome; again, the mother was later found to have mosaic Down's syndrome. It may be significant that both these mothers were born when their own mothers were 39 years old. Theoretically, a similar situation could occur with a father who had a low degree of mosaicism. While these instances of parents with some degree of mosaicism may be interesting from a biological point of view, *they are rare and therefore are probably not of great importance* when giving an overall consideration of how Down's syndrome occurs. However, it is of great importance to individual parents who are affected when they are considering the risk of Down's syndrome occurring in future births.

As you may well have gathered, it is not always easy to diagnose mosaic Down's syndrome. For instance, an individual's blood may be free of abnormal cells, yet trisomic cells may be found in skin, or blood and skin may be almost free of abnormal cells, yet the ovaries may have a high percentage of trisomic cells. The situation can be further complicated when *translocation* is involved in the affected cell line (translocation is explained later).

How does mosaic Down's syndrome occur?

As we have noted, mosaicism occurs when different groups of cells (or cell lines) within an individual have different numbers of chromosomes. In mosaic Down's syndrome this usually means that some cells have 46 chromosomes, and are normal, but others have trisomy 21 and therefore have 47 chromosomes.

However, the first report of mosaicism in humans actually involved an anomaly of the sex chromosomes, known as Kleinfelter's syndrome. This occurs in males when they have one (or perhaps more) extra X chromosomes, and the individual involved here had an extra X chromosome in some of his cells. To confuse the issue further, the man affected also had full Down's syndrome, so all his cells had an extra number 21 chromosome as well. This first report was published in 1959, but two years later an American research team reported a case where mosaic Down's syndrome was involved, i.e. some cells were normal and some had trisomy 21. A week later another case was reported in Britain, and several other cases were published during the following twelve months. Yet the fact remains that mosaicism is a comparatively rare form of Down's syndrome.

In terms of biology, mosaic Down's syndrome may arise by three basic mechanisms.

(i) Normal zygote non-disjunction
In this case a normal egg and sperm fuse to form a normal zygote. It is only when the zygote starts to divide by the usual process of mitosis that the problem arises; chromosome pair number 21 failing to separate properly during the second or subsequent cell divisions. Hence we may say that non-disjunction has occurred during mitosis in a normal zygote (see right-hand diagram, Figure 10). It has been estimated that only about 1 in 160,000 births that started off as normal fertilized eggs would be affected by this type of non-disjunction.

Interestingly enough, if non-disjunction occurred at the very first mitotic division of the zygote, then the baby would have full trisomy

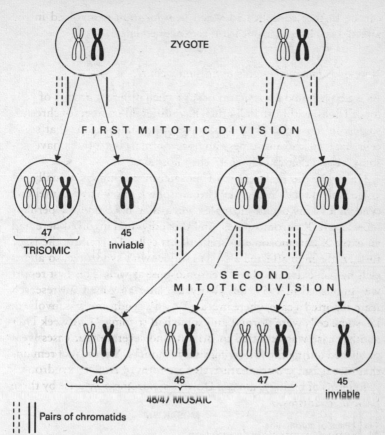

Figure 10. Non-disjunction a normal zygote. (If this process occurs at the first mitotic division of a normal zygote then full trisomy results, but if it occurs at the second mitotic division then 46/47 mosaicism results.)

21, as the cell with only 45 chromosomes would die (see left-hand diagram, Figure 10).

(ii) Trisomic zygote anaphase lagging

In this situation we start off with a trisomic zygote that has arisen because either egg or sperm has an extra chromosome 21 (see: *Trisomy 21, Non-disjunction and Down's syndrome*, page 166).

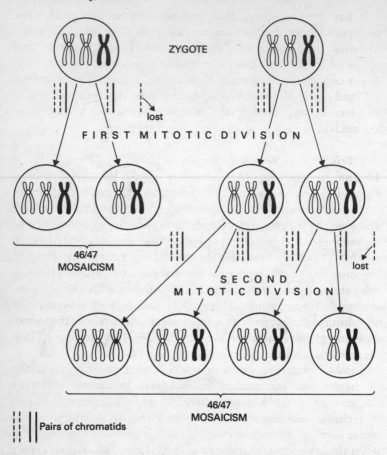

ZYGOTE

lost

FIRST MITOTIC DIVISION

46/47
MOSAICISM

SECOND
MITOTIC DIVISION

lost

46/47
MOSAICISM

Pairs of chromatids

Figure 11. Diagram showing the results of anaphase lagging in a trisomic zygote at first and second mitotic divisions. (46/47 mosaicism results whether this process occurs at the first or second mitotic division of a trisomic zygote.)

This zygote then starts to divide by the usual method of mitosis. The chromosomes split longitudinally, but at a certain stage one half (or chromatid) of number 21 chromosomes does not move properly to the correct place in the dividing cell, and is therefore lost to the cell during division. This process results in some cells having 46 chromosomes and some having 47, whether it occurs at the first or at subsequent cell divisions (see Figure 11).

It has been suggested that trisomic zygotes are much more susceptible to events resulting in mosaicism than normal zygotes. Richards, the scientist who made this observation, suggested that out of all the mosaic Down's syndrome population, probably only 20 per cent would have arisen from normal zygotes (i.e. by method (i)), and nearly 80 per cent would have come from trisomic zygote anaphase lagging. The few remaining may have arisen by the following mechanism:

(iii) Trisomic zygote non-disjunction

This mechanism seems to be very rare indeed. Initially, a trisomic zygote is formed because either the egg or the sperm contains an extra chromosome. However, during one of the subsequent cell divisions the trisomic zygote undergoes non-disjunction of one of its number 21 chromosomes. Hence one resulting cell loses a number 21 chromosome and the other gains yet another extra 21 chromosome. If this happens at the first cell division, then two cell lines are produced; one containing 46 chromosomes and one containing 48 chromosomes. This may be called 46/48 mosaicism. If non-disjunction happens at a subsequent cell division, then three different cell lines will be produced (i.e. 46/47/48 mosaicism). These two eventualities are represented in Figure 12.

Another interesting aspect of mosaicism is that there is evidence to suggest that the ratio of trisomic cells to normal cells may change over a period of time. Research has shown that this ratio may change in either direction, giving either an increase or a decrease in the proportion of trisomic cells. It has been suggested that when the proportion of trisomic cells increases, the original zygote may have been trisomic, while the original zygote may have been normal when the proportion of trisomic cells decreases. In fact, drastic changes in the proportions of different cell lines may occur before birth, or even in laboratory cell cultures, and this can make it very difficult to establish how the mosaicism arose. For instance, if a cell line with 48 chromosomes was lost after the rare trisomic zygote non-disjunction, then the resulting baby would appear to have 46/47 mosaicism. Consequently genetic investigation of the cells would tend to indicate that the apparently more common mechanism of trisomic zygote anaphase lagging had occurred.

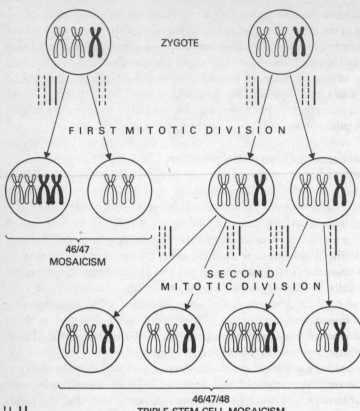

ZYGOTE

FIRST MITOTIC DIVISION

46/47
MOSAICISM

SECOND
MITOTIC DIVISION

|| ||| Pairs of chromatids

46/47/48
TRIPLE STEM CELL MOSAICISM

Figure 12. Diagram showing the results of non-disjunction in a trisomic zygote. (If non-disjunction occurs in a trisomic zygote at the first mitotic division, 46/47 mosaicism results; if it occurs at the second mitotic division 46/47/48 mosaicism results.)

Furthermore, when genetic tests are done and tissue samples are grown *in vitro*, they may not behave as they do *in vivo*; different cell lines may divide at different rates – some may not even survive. Therefore the ratio of normal to trisomic cells found in tissue cultures from people with mosaic Down's syndrome cannot be reliably used to indicate the particular division at which the error took place.

To complete the picture of mosaic Down's syndrome, a classification of the different types of mosaicism should be mentioned. Mosaicism tends not to be classified by the mechanism from which it arises (as described in (i) – (iii) above), but rather by the extent and type of involvement of trisomic cells in the body tissues. Three types of mosaicism may be identified:

(a) Cellular mosaicism

This is the most common form of mosaicism, where a single tissue may contain both normal cells and trisomic cells. This could theoretically arise from any of the mechanisms which have been discussed.

(b) Tissue mosaicism

This is a rare situation where specific tissues are affected by trisomy 21. In this type of mosaicism, for instance, certain white blood cells may show a single trisomic cell line, while a particular group of skin cells may appear entirely normal.

(c) Chimerism

This is again very rare. In this situation two separately fertilized eggs fuse together to grow into a single individual. Because two separate eggs are involved it cannot strictly be considered to be a true form of mosaicism. A person with *chimerism* would not necessarily have to have any trisomic cells, although clearly if that person was affected by Down's syndrome, one or both ova would have some form of trisomy for chromosome 21. The first chimeric case of Down's syndrome to be reported presented a ratio of 4:1 normal to trisomy 21 cells in blood cultures and complete trisomy 21 in a particular type of skin cell culture. Further biochemical analysis enabled the researchers to identify two genetically distinct blood cell populations; hence two products of conception must have fused to form a single individual.

Of course, the type of mosaicism involved or the method by which it arose makes little difference to the individual affected, and is not apparent from appearance.

What is translocation?

We have so far said that people with Down's syndrome have a complete extra number 21 chromosome in some or all of their cells. Is this always the case?

Following the discovery by Lejeune of the extra chromosome in people with Down's syndrome, a surge of interest was generated in chromosomal analysis of the condition. It was while investigating three children with Down's syndrome who had been born to quite young mothers that Polani and his colleagues at Guy's Hospital found that one of these children seemed to have the normal comple- ment of 46 chromosomes. Yet the child in question still had all the typical features of Down's syndrome. Further detailed analysis still revealed only a single pair of number 21 chromosomes, but chromo- some number 14 seemed to be unusually long. After more investig- ation it was decided that the extra material on chromosome 14 consisted of part of another number 21 chromosome. In other words, part of an extra chromosome 21 had joined to a chromo- some 14, and the rest of the extra 21 chromosome had been lost. This meant that certain areas of chromosome 21 were present in triplic- ate in this child. When part of one chromosome joins to another in this fashion it is referred to as a *translocation* (see Figure 13).

This was the first report of translocation in Down's syndrome involving *non-homologous* chromosomes (i.e. not from the same pair), although interestingly enough a chromosome re-arrangement had been suggested by Lionel Penrose about fifty years ago as one possible explanation for Down's syndrome.

Immediately following Polani's paper in the *Lancet* there ap- peared the first report of a translocation between two *homologous* chromosomes (i.e. from the same pair). The cytogenetic findings in this case showed one normal 21 and one unusually long 21. It became clear that what had happened was that the extra 21 had become attached to one of the other chromosomes in the number 21 pair.

The translocations causing Down's syndrome usually happen either between chromosome groups D and G, or within chromo- some group G. They are therefore known as D/G or G/G transloca- tions respectively.

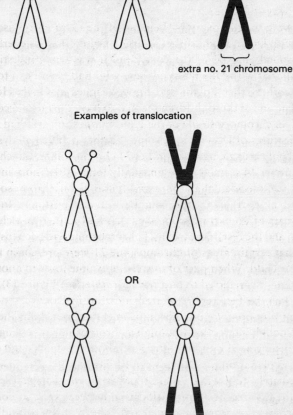

Figure 13. Trisomy 21 compared with examples of translocation.

From the point of view of the individual with Down's syndrome, it is of course of little importance to clarify whether the Down's syndrome has occurred because of standard trisomy or because of translocation; especially as it seems to make no difference to the subsequent development of the child, and because translocation only accounts for around 5 or 6 per cent of the total population with Down's syndrome. Yet in terms of advising families with an affected child as to the possibility of conceiving further children with Down's syndrome, the type of chromosomal arrangement is of great importance.

Translocations may either be inherited, or may arise spontaneously. In the case of inherited translocations, either parent can be the carrier. That is, though the carrier parent is completely normal in all other respects, he or she appears to have only 45 chromosomes. In reality the 'missing' 21 chromosome is attached elsewhere in the same way as the *extra* chromosome is in a person with translocation Down's syndrome.

While still remaining rare, the most common D/G translocation appearing in Down's syndrome is between chromosomes 14 and 21. If one parent carries this translocation it means that the theoretical chances of conceiving a child with Down's syndrome would be as high as one in three. In practice it works out at about one in six or seven live births if it is the mother that carries the translocation. If it is the father, the chances may be less; about one in twenty. While again still rare, a G/G translocation in Down's syndrome is usually between two number 21 chromosomes. If one parent carries this translocation it would mean that all live births would be affected by Down's syndrome.

It would seem, therefore, with inherited D/G translocations, that the chances of passing the translocation on are higher if the mother is the carrier. One explanation put forward for this has been that the affected sperm does not seem to be produced as frequently as theoretically expected, or it has either a lower survival rate up to fertilization or a lower fertilization potential for some reason.

Spontaneous, or *de novo* translocations can also happen. In this situation neither parent is a carrier, as the translocation happens spontaneously during the formation of eggs or sperms. In this case the high risk of having another child with Down's syndrome would not be expected to exist, although the risk may not be quite as low as for parents who had never had any children with Down's syndrome.

It is important to stress that when considering the frequency of any type of Down's syndrome births, the figures quoted are most unlikely to reflect conception incidences. There will be a considerable number of foetuses lost before birth, and it is likely that the rate of loss of foetuses with Down's syndrome is higher than that of unaffected foetuses. Furthermore, the rate of loss of foetuses with different sorts of Down's syndrome, or even different sorts of translocations, may well not be the same.

Of course, much greater detail is known about the biology of Down's syndrome than is included here. However, this Appendix will hopefully serve as an introduction to the interested reader. For those wanting a fuller explanation, current medical texts should be consulted.

REFERENCES

Alberman, E., Polani, P. E., Fraser Roberts, J. A., Spicer, C. C., Elliott, M., and Armstrong, E. (1972): 'Parental exposure to X-irradiation and Down's syndrome', *Annals of Human Genetics*, 36, 195–202.

Atkin, J., and Goode, J. (1982): 'Learning at home and at school', *Education*, 20, 3–13.

Bleyer, A. (1934): 'Indication that mongoloid imbecility is a genetic mutation of the degressive type', *American Journal of Diseases in Children*, 47, 342–8.

Blumberg, B. S., Gerstley, B. J. S., Sutrick, A. I., Millman, I., and London, W. T. (1970): 'Australia antigen, hepatitis virus and Down's Syndrome'. *Annals of the New York Academy of Science*, 171, 486.

Book, J. A., Fraccaro, M., and Lindsten, J. (1959): 'Cytogenetical observations in mongolism', *Acta paediatrica*, 48, 453.

Brinkworth, R. (1985): 'Possibilities and achievements', in D. Lane and B. Stratford, *Current Approaches to Down's Syndrome*. Eastbourne: Holt, Rinehard & Winston.

Brothers, C. R. D., and Jago, G. C. (1954): 'Report on the longevity and the cause of death in mongoloidism in the State of Victoria', *Journal of Mental Science*, 100, 580.

Brothwell, D. R. (1960): 'A possible case of Mongolism in a Saxon population', *Annals of Human Genetics*, 24, 141–7.

Carter, C. O. (1958): 'A life table for mongols with causes of death', *Journal of Mental Deficiency Research*, 2, 64–7.

Carter, C. O., Evans, K. A., and Stewart, A. M. (1961): 'Maternal radiation and Down's syndrome', *Lancet*, 1042.

Chambers, R. (1844): *The Vestiges of the Natural History of Creation*. London: Churchill.

Chu, E. H. Y., and Giles, N. H. (1959): 'Human chromosome complements in normal somatic cells in culture', *American Journal of Human Genetics*, 11, 63–78.

Clarke, R. M. (1929): 'The mongol – a new explanation', *Journal of Mental*

Science, 75, 261–4.

Cohen, B. H., Likenfeld, A. M., Kramer, S., and Hyman, L. C. (1977): 'Parental factors in Down's syndrome – results of the second Baltimore case-control study', in E. B. Hook and I. H. Porter (eds.), *Population Cytogenetics. Studies in Humans.* New York: Academic Press.

Collman, R. D., and Stoller, A. (1963): 'A life table for mongols in Victoria, Australia', *Journal of Mental Deficiency Research,* 7, 60.

Comas, J. (1942): 'El problema de la existencia de un tipo racial olmeca', Sociedad Mexicana de Antropologia Reninones de Mesa Redonda, *Mayas y Olmecas,* 69–70.

Covarrubias, M. (1946): 'El arte "Olmec" o de la Venta', *Cuadernos Americanos,* 4, 153–79.

Covarrubias, M. (1957): *Indian Art of Mexico and Central America.* New York: Knopf.

Cranefield, P. E., and Ferdern, W. (1967): 'Paracelsus: The Begetting of Fools', *Bulletin of the History of Medicine,* 41, 56–63.

Crookshank, F. G. (1924): *The Mongol in our Midst.* London: Kegan Paul.

Cullen, J. F., and Butler, H. G. (1963): 'Down's Syndrome and Keratoconus', *British Journal of Ophthalmics,* 47, 321–5.

Deaton, J. G. (1973): 'The mortality rate and causes of death among institutionalised mongols in Texas', *Journal of Mental Deficiency Research,* 17, 117–20.

Down, J. L. H. (1866): 'Observations on an ethnic classification of idiots', *London Hospital Clinical Lectures and Reports,* 3, 259.

Down, J. L. H. (1887): *On Some of the Mental Afflictions of Childhood and Youth.* London: Churchill.

Duffy, L., and Wishart, J. G. (1987): 'A comparison of two procedures for teaching discrimination skills to Down's syndrome and non-handicapped children', *British Journal of Educational Psychology,* 57, 265–78.

Eden, D. J. (1976): *Mental Handicap – An Introduction.* London: Allen & Unwin.

Esquirol, J. E. D. (1838): *Des Maladies Mentales sous les Rapports Médical, Hygiénique et Médico-legal,* 2 vols. Paris: Baillière.

Fabia, J., and Drolette, M. (1970): 'Life tables up to age 10 for mongols with and without congenital heart defects', *Journal of Mental Deficiency Research,* 14, 235–9.

Ford, C. E., and Hamerton, J. L. (1956): 'The chromosomes of man', *Nature,* 168, 1020–26.

Frazer, J., and Mitchell, A. (1876): 'Kalmuc idiocy: report on a case with autopsy and notes on 62 cases', *Journal of Mental Science,* 22, 169–72.

Gardiner, P. A. (1967): 'Visual defects in cases of Down's syndrome and in other mentally handicapped children', *British Journal of Ophthalmology*, 51, 469.

Greene-Robertson, M., Rosenblum-Scandizzo, M. S., and Scandizzo, J. R. (1974): 'Physical deformities in the ruling lineage of Palenque and the dynastic implications', in *The Art, Iconography and Dynastic History of Palenque*, Part III: The proceedings of the Segunda Mesa Redonda de Palenque, M. Greene-Robertson (ed), pp. 59–86. Pebble Beach: Pre-Columbian Art Research, Robert Louis Stevenson School.

Hallidie-Smith, K. A. (1985): 'The Heart', in D. Lane and B. Stratford, *Current Approaches to Down's Syndrome*. Eastbourne: Holt, Rinehart & Winston.

Hanson, E. (1985): *Parental Perceptions of Professionals*. M.Ed. dissertation, University of Nottingham.

Harrell, H. F., Capp, R. H., Davis, D. R., Peerless, J., and Ravitz, L. R. (1981): 'Can nutritional supplements help mentally retarded children? An exploratory study', *Proceedings of the National Academy of Science USA*, 78, 574–8.

Hutchinson, J. (1886): 'Some moot points on the natural history of syphilis', *British Medical Journal*, 1, 22.

Jenkins, R. L. (1933): 'Etiology of mongolism', *American Journal of Diseases in Children*, 45, 506.

Kirman, B. (1975): 'Historical and legal aspects', in B. Kirman and J. Bicknell, *Mental Handicap*. London: Churchill Livingstone.

Lejeune, J., Gautier, M., and Turpin, R. (1959a): 'Les chromosomes humains en culture de tissus', *Comptes Rendus Hebdomanaires des Séances de l'Académie des Sciences*, 248, 602–3.

Lejeune, J., Gautier, M., and Turpin, R. (1959b): 'Études des chromosomes somatiques de neuf enfants mongoliens', *Comptes Rendus Hebdomanaires des Séances de l'Académie des Sciences*, 248, 1721–2.

Lunn, J. E. (1959): 'A survey of mongol children in Glasgow', *Scottish Medical Journal*, 4, 368–72.

Marmol, J. G., Scriggins, A. L., and Vollman, R. F. (1969): 'Mothers of mongoloid infants in the collaborative project', *American Journal of Obstetrics and Gynaecology*, 533–43.

Mavor, J. W. (1922): 'The production of non-disjunction by X-rays', *Science*, 55, 295–7.

Mavor, J. W. (1924): 'The production of non-disjunction by X-rays', *Journal of Experimental Zoology*, 39, 382–432.

McDonald, A. D. (1972): 'Thyroid disease and other material factors in mongolism', *Canadian Medical Association Journal, 160,* 1085–92.

Meyers, C. R. (1938): 'An application of the control method of the problem of the etiology of mongolism', *American Association of Mental Deficiency,* Proceedings of the 62nd Annual Session, *43,* 142.

Milton, G., and Gonzalo, R. (1974): 'Jaguar Cult — Down's Syndrome — Were — Jaguar', *Expedition, 16,* 33–7.

Mittler, P., and Mittler, H. (1982): *Partnership with Parents.* National Council for Special Education.

Mittler, P. (1979): 'Patterns of partnership between parents and professionals', *Parents Voice, 29.*

Mittwoch, U. (1952): 'The chromosome complement in a mongolian imbecile', *Annals of Eugenics, 17,* 37–81.

Murdoch, J. C. (1985): *The Down's Family Project.* University of Otago, New Zealand.

Painter, T. S. (1921): 'The Y chromosome in mammals', *Science, 53,* 503.

Patterson, J. T., Brewster, W., and Winchester, A. M. (1932): 'Effects produced by ageing and X-raying eggs of Drosophila Melanogaster', *Journal of Heredity, 32,* 325–33.

Penrose, L. S. (1932): 'On the interaction of heredity and environment in the study of human genetics, with special reference to mongolian imbecility', *Journal of Genetics, 25,* 407.

Penrose, L. S. (1949): 'The incidence of mongolism in the general population', *Journal of Mental Science, 95,* 685.

Reich, S. G. (1979): *Pathology in Olmec Art.* Degree thesis, Department of Latin American Studies, Tulane University.

Richards, B. W., and Sylvester, P. E. (1969): 'Mortality trends in mental deficiency institutions', *Journal of Mental Deficiency Research, 15,* 276.

Rollin, H. R. (1946): 'Personality in mongolism with special reference to the incidence of catatonic psychosis', *American Journal of Mental Deficiency, 51,* 219–37.

Ryan, J., and Thomas, F. (1981): 'Mental handicap: the historical background', in W. Swann (ed.), *The Practice of Special Education.* Open University. Oxford: Blackwell.

Séguin, E. (1846): *Le traitement moral, l'hygiène et l'éducation des idiots.* Paris: Baillière.

Séguin, E. (1866): *Idiocy and its Treatment by the Psychological Method.* New York: Wood.

Sewell, G. (1981): 'The micro-sociology of segregation', in L. Barton and S. Tomlinson (eds.), *Special Education: Policy, Practices and Social Issues.* Harper & Row.

Sheehan, P. M. E., and Hillary, I. B. (1983): 'An unusual cluster of babies with Down's syndrome born to former pupils of an Irish boarding school', *British Medical Journal, 287*, 1428–9.

Sheehan, P. M. E., and Hillary, I. B. (1984): 'An unusual cluster of babies with Down's Syndrome', *British Medical Journal, 288*, 147–8.

Shuttleworth, G. E. (1866): 'Clinical lecture on idiocy and imbecility', *British Medical Journal, 1*, 183–8.

Shuttleworth, G. E. (1906): 'Comments on J. L. Down's paper', *Journal of Mental Science, 52*, 189.

Shuttleworth, G. E. (1909): 'Mongolian imbecility', *British Medical Journal, 2*, 661–3.

Sigler, A. T., Lilienfeld, A. M., Cohen, B. H., and Westlake, J. E. (1965): 'Radiation exposure in parents of children with Down's Syndrome', *Bulletin of the Johns Hopkins Hospital, 117*, 374–99.

Smith, G. F., and Berg, J. M. (1976): *Down's Anomaly*, 2nd edn. London and New York: Churchill Livingstone.

Stevenson, A. C., Mason, R., and Edwards, K. D. (1970): 'Maternal diagnostic X-irradiation before conception and the frequency of mongolism in children subsequently born', *Lancet*, 1335–7.

Stevenson, A. C., and Matousek, V. (1961): *United Nations Document A/AC82/G/L700*.

Stott, D. H. (1961): 'Mongolism related to emotional shock in early pregnancy', *Vita Hum (Basel), 4*, 57–61.

Stratford, B. (1982): 'Down's syndrome at the Court of Mantua', *Journal of Family Medicine: Maternal and Child Health, 7*, 250–54.

Stratford, B., and Au, M. L. (1988): 'The development of drawing in Chinese and English children', *Early Child Development and Care, 30*, 141–65.

Stratford, B., and Ching, E. Y. Y. (1983): 'Rhythm and time in the perception of Down's syndrome children', *Journal of Mental Deficiency Research, 27*, 23–38.

Stratford, B., and Ching, E. Y. Y. (1989): 'Music and movement in the development of children with Down's syndrome', *Journal of Mental Deficiency Research* (in press).

Stratford, B., and Steele, J. (1985): 'Incidence and prevalence of Down's Syndrome', *Journal of Mental Deficiency Research, 29*, 95–107.

Sutherland, G. A. (1899): 'Mongolian imbecility in infants', *Practitioner, 63*, 632–5.

Sutherland, G. A. (1900): 'Differential diagnosis of mongolism and cretinism', *Lancet, 1*, 23.

Thase, M. E. (1982): 'Reversible dementia in Down's syndrome', *Journal of Mental Deficiency Research, 26,* 111–13.

Tijo, J. H., and Puck, T. T. (1958): 'The somatic chromosomes of man', *Proceedings of the National Academy of Science USA, 44,* 1229–37.

Tijo, J. H., and Levan, A. (1956): 'The chromosome number of man', *Hereditas, 42,* 1–4.

Uchida, I. A., and Curtis, E. J. (1961): 'A possible association between maternal radiation and mongolism', *Lancet, 2,* 848–50.

Uchida, I. A., Holunga, R., and Lawler, C. (1968): 'Maternal radiation and chromosomal aberrations', *Lancet,* 1045–9.

United Nations (1982): *Report of the United Nations Scientific Committee on the Effects of Atomic Radiation. Official Records of the 37th Session, Supplement No. 45 (A/37/45).* New York: United Nations.

Waardenburg, P. J. (1932): *Das menschliche Aug und Seine Erbanlagen.* The Hague: Nijhoff.

Wald, N., Turner, J. H., and Borges, W. (1970): 'Down's syndrome and exposure to X-irradiation', *Annals of the New York Academy of Science, 171,* 454–66.

Weathers, C. (1983): 'Effects of nutritional supplementation on IQ and certain other variables associated with Down's Syndrome', *American Journal of Mental Deficiency, 88,* 214–17.

Weihs, T. J. (1977): *In Need of Special Care.* First Annual Segal Lecture: Leeds University.

Wicke, C. P. (1971): *Olmec: An Early Style of Pre-Columbian Mexico.* Tucson: University of Arizona Press.

Winiwarters, H. von (1912): 'Études sur la spermatogenèse humaine', *Archives de Biologie, 27,* 91–189.

Zellweger, H. (1968): 'Is Down's syndrome a modern disease?', *Lancet, 2,* 458–61.

FURTHER READING

Medical and technical

Gibson, D. (1978): *Down's Syndrome: the psychology of mongolism*. Cambridge: Cambridge University Press.

Pueschel, S. M., and Rynders, J. E. (1982): *Down's Syndrome: Advances in Biomedicine and the Behavioural Sciences*. New York: Ware Press.

Smith, G. F., and Berg, J. M. (1976): *Down's Anomaly* (2nd edn). London and New York: Churchill Livingstone.

Professional

(but also suitable in style and content for parents and the general reader who is seeking more technical and detailed information)

Carr, J. (1975): *Young Children with Down's Syndrome*. London: Butterworth.

Gath, A. (1978): *Down's Syndrome and the Family: the early years*. London: Academic Press.

Lane, D., and Stratford, B. (1987): *Current Approaches to Down's Syndrome* (2nd imp.). London: Cassell.

Pueschel, S. M. (1984): *The Young Child with Down's Syndrome*. New York: Human Sciences Press.

Pueschel, S. M. et al. (1987): *New Perspectives on Down's Syndrome*. New York: Brookes.

A selection of books for parents and the general reader

Information about these and other books, booklets and pamphlets on Down's syndrome is available from the Down's Syndrome Association and the Royal Society for Mentally Handicapped Children and Adults. Lists will be supplied by these organizations on application.

Examples of the kind of titles available

A useful series from Souvenir Press under such titles as *Let me Read, Let me Speak, Learning to Cope, Let me Play*, etc.

Carr, J. (1980): *Helping Your Handicapped Child*. Harmondsworth: Penguin Books.

Craft, A., and Craft, M. (1983): *Sex Education and Counselling for Mentally Handicapped People*. Tunbridge Wells: Costello.

Craft, M., and Craft, A. (1979): *Sex and the Mentally Handicapped*. London: Routledge & Kegan Paul.

Cunningham, C. C. (1982): *Down's Syndrome – An introduction for parents*. London: Souvenir Press.

Cunningham, C. C., and Sloper, P. (1978): *Helping Your Handicapped Baby*. London: Souvenir Press.

Furneaux, B. (1981): *The Special Child*. Harmondsworth: Penguin Books, 3rd edn.

Hewitt, S. (1970): *The Family and the Handicapped Child*. London: Allen & Unwin.

Tingey, C. (1988): *Down's Syndrome*. Taylor & Francis.

McClintock, A. B. (1981): *Drama for Mentally Handicapped Children*. London: Souvenir Press.

Wood, M. (1983): *Music for Mentally Handicapped People*. London: Souvenir Press.

Books and other publications from the Portsmouth Down's Syndrome Trust:

The proceeds of all these publications supports the work of the Trust. They are available only from:

> The Portsmouth Down's Syndrome Trust
> Psychology Department
> Portsmouth Polytechnic
> King Charles Street
> Portsmouth PO1 2ER

Buckley, S., et al.: *The Development of Language and Reading Skills in Children with Down's Syndrome*.

Buckley, S., and Sacks, B.: *The Adolescent with Down's Syndrome – Life for the teenager and for the family*.

Two useful videotapes are also available from the Portsmouth Down's Syndrome Trust:

Reading skills in children with Down's syndrome is a 35-minute tape showing methods of early reading. A 60-minute tape is also available which illustrates the development of language and reading skills.

SOME USEFUL ADDRESSES

For literature, advice or any information concerning Down's syndrome in Great Britain:

> **Down's Syndrome Association**
> **12–13 Clapham Common Southside**
> **London SW4 7AA**

Software for Micromate computer system (page 126):

> **Toys for the Handicapped**
> **Micromate Software**
> **Stourport**
> **Hereford and Worcester**

Further information on Computer Assisted Learning (page 127):

> **The Vocational and Rehabilitation Research Institute**
> **3304 33rd Street, N.W.**
> **Calgary**
> **Alberta T2L 2A6**
> **Canada**

For all kinds of information and literature on mental handicap generally:

> **The Royal Society for Mentally Handicapped Children and Adults (MENCAP)**
> **123 Golden Lane**
> **London EC1Y 0RT**

Travelling abroad?

Parents are sometimes worried about local or national regulations concerning health, insurance and immigration restrictions when travelling overseas with children with Down's syndrome. Information can be obtained from the following addresses:

USA

> Downs Syndrome Congress
> 1640 W. Roosevelt Road
> Chicago, IL 60608

EUROPE

> European Down's Syndrome Association
> c/o Department of Psychology
> University of Liège
> Belgium

HONG KONG

> HKDSA
> 26 Peak Road 1/F
> Cheung Chau Island
> Hong Kong

Other Far Eastern Countries

> General Secretary
> HKASSMH
> c/o 11 Renfrew Road
> Kowloon Tong
> Hong Kong

LATIN AMERICA

> ALASD
> Boulevard de la Luz 232
> Jardine del Pedregal
> 01900 Mexico, D.F.

ZIMBABWE
   Zimbabwe Down's Children's Association
   P.O. Box 5706
   Harare
   Zimbabwe

(This very active Association can provide information about other African countries.)

AUSTRALIA
   Down's Syndrome Research Unit
   Fred and Eleanor Schonell Research Centre
   University of Queensland
   Australia

INDIA
   Professor I. C. Verma
   Department of Paediatrics
   All India Institute of Medical Sciences
   New Delhi
   India

For contacts in other areas apply to **Down's Syndrome Association, Great Britain** (address on page 189).

Index

NOTE: Down's syndrome is abbreviated to DS.

FOR THE BEST IN PAPERBACKS, LOOK FOR THE

In every corner of the world, on every subject under the sun, Penguin represents quality and variety – the very best in publishing today.

For complete information about books available from Penguin – including Puffins, Penguin Classics and Arkana – and how to order them, write to us at the appropriate address below. Please note that for copyright reasons the selection of books varies from country to country.

In the United Kingdom: Please write to *Dept E.P., Penguin Books Ltd, Harmondsworth, Middlesex, UB7 0DA.*

If you have any difficulty in obtaining a title, please send your order with the correct money, plus ten per cent for postage and packaging, to *PO Box No 11, West Drayton, Middlesex*

In the United States: Please write to *Dept BA, Penguin, 299 Murray Hill Parkway, East Rutherford, New Jersey 07073*

In Canada: Please write to *Penguin Books Canada Ltd, 2801 John Street, Markham, Ontario L3R 1B4*

In Australia: Please write to the *Marketing Department, Penguin Books Australia Ltd, P.O. Box 257, Ringwood, Victoria 3134*

In New Zealand: Please write to the *Marketing Department, Penguin Books (NZ) Ltd, Private Bag, Takapuna, Auckland 9*

In India: Please write to *Penguin Overseas Ltd, 706 Eros Apartments, 56 Nehru Place, New Delhi, 110019*

In the Netherlands: Please write to *Penguin Books Netherlands B.V., Postbus 195, NL–1380AD Weesp*

In West Germany: Please write to *Penguin Books Ltd, Friedrichstrasse 10–12, D–6000 Frankfurt/Main 1*

In Spain: Please write to *Alhambra Longman S.A.; Fernandez de la Hoz 9, E–28010 Madrid*

In Italy: Please write to *Penguin Italia s.r.l., Via Como 4, 1-20096 Pioltello (Milano)*

In France: Please write to *Penguin Books Ltd, 39 Rue de Montmorency, F-75003 Paris*

In Japan: Please write to *Longman Penguin Japan Co Ltd, Yamaguchi Building, 2-12-9 Kanda Jimbocho, Chiyoda-Ku, Tokyo 101*

A CHOICE OF PENGUINS

Brian Epstein: The Man Who Made the Beatles   Ray Coleman

'An excellent biography of Brian Epstein, the lonely, gifted man whose artistic faith and bond with the Beatles never wavered – and whose recognition of genius created a cultural era, even though it destroyed him' – *Mail on Sunday*

A Thief in the Night   John Cornwell

A veil of suspicion and secrecy surrounds the last hours of Pope John Paul I, whose thirty-three day reign ended in a reported heart attack on the night of 28 September 1978. Award-winning crime writer John Cornwell was invited by the Vatican to investigate. 'The best detective story you will ever read' – *Daily Mail*

Among the Russians   Colin Thubron

One man's solitary journey by car across Russia provides an enthralling and revealing account of the habits and idiosyncrasies of a fascinating people. 'He sees things with the freshness of an innocent and the erudition of a scholar' – *Daily Telegraph*

Higher than Hope   Fatima Meer

The authorized biography of Nelson Mandela. 'An astonishing read ... the most complete, authoritative and moving tribute thus far' – *Time Out*

Stones of Aran: Pilgrimage   Tim Robinson

Arainn is the largest of the three Aran Islands, and one of the world's oldest landscapes. This 'wholly irresistible' (*Observer*) and uncategorizable book charts a sunwise journey around its coast – and explores an open secret, teasing out the paradoxes of a terrain at once bare and densely inscribed.

Bernard Shaw   Michael Holroyd
Volume I 1856–1898: The Search for Love

'In every sense, a spectacular piece of work ... A feat of style as much as of research, which will surely make it a flamboyant new landmark in modern English life-writing' – Richard Holmes in *The Times*

A CHOICE OF PENGUINS

Return to the Marshes Gavin Young

His remarkable portrait of the remote and beautiful world of the Marsh Arabs, whose centuries-old existence is now threatened with extinction by twentieth-century warfare.

The Big Red Train Ride Eric Newby

From Moscow to the Pacific on the Trans-Siberian Railway is an eight-day journey of nearly six thousand miles through seven time zones. In 1977 Eric Newby set out with his wife, an official guide and a photographer on this journey.

Warhol Victor Bockris

'This is the kind of book I like: it tells me the things I want to know about the artist, what he ate, what he wore, who he knew (in his case ... everybody), at what time he went to bed and with whom, and, most important of all, his work habits' – *Independent*

1001 Ways to Save the Planet Bernadette Vallely

There are 1001 changes that *everyone* can make in their lives *today* to bring about a greener environment – whether at home or at work, on holiday or away on business. Action that you can take *now*, and that you won't find too difficult to take. This practical guide shows you how.

Bitter Fame Anne Stevenson
A Life of Sylvia Plath

'A sobering and salutary attempt to estimate what Plath was, what she achieved and what it cost her ... This is the only portrait which answers Ted Hughes's image of the poet as Ariel, not the ethereal bright pure roving sprite, but Ariel trapped in Prospero's pine and raging to be free' – *Sunday Telegraph*

The Venetian Empire Jan Morris

For six centuries the Republic of Venice was a maritime empire of coasts, islands and fortresses. Jan Morris reconstructs this glittering dominion in the form of a sea voyage along the historic Venetian trade routes from Venice itself to Greece, Crete and Cyprus.

FOR THE BEST IN PAPERBACKS, LOOK FOR THE

A CHOICE OF PENGUINS

Trail of Havoc Patrick Marnham

The murder of the 7th Earl of Lucan's nanny at the family's Belgravia mansion in 1974 remains one of the most celebrated mysteries in British criminal history. In this brilliant piece of detective work Patrick Marnham investigates the Lucan case and its implications and arrives at some surprising conclusions: what was not disclosed at the murder inquest and what probably *did* happen on that fateful night.

Daddy, We Hardly Knew You Germaine Greer

'It's part biography, part travelogue, its author obsessively scouring three continents for clues to her dead father's identity ... ruthlessly stripping away the ornate masks with which [he] hid his own flawed humanity' – *Time Out*. 'Remarkable, beautifully written' – Anthony Storr

Reports from the holocaust Larry Kramer

'Larry Kramer is one of America's most valuable troublemakers. I hope he never lowers his voice' – Susan Sontag. It was Larry Kramer who first fought to make America aware – notably in his play *The Normal Heart* – of the scope of the AIDS epidemic. 'More than a political autobiography, *Reports* is an indictment of a world that allows AIDS to continue' – *Newsday*

A Far Cry Mary Benson

'A remarkable life, bravely lived ... A lovely book and a piece of history' – Nadine Gordimer. 'One of those rare autobiographies which can tell a moving personal story and illuminate a public political drama. It recounts the South African battles against apartheid with a new freshness and intimacy' – *Observer*

The Fate of the Forest Susanna Hecht and Alexander Cockburn

In a panorama that encompasses history, ecology, botany and economics, *The Fate of the Forest* tells the story of the delusions and greed that have shaped the Amazon's history – and shows how it can be saved. 'This discriminating and constructive book is a must' – *Sunday Times*

A CHOICE OF PENGUINS

Citizens Simon Schama

'The most marvellous book I have read about the French Revolution in the last fifty years' – Richard Cobb in *The Times*. 'He has chronicled the vicissitudes of that world with matchless understanding, wisdom, pity and truth, in the pages of this huge and marvellous book' – *Sunday Times*

Out of Africa Karen Blixen (Isak Dinesen)

After the failure of her coffee-farm in Kenya, where she lived from 1913 to 1931, Karen Blixen went home to Denmark and wrote this unforgettable account of her experiences. 'No reader can put the book down without some share in the author's poignant farewell to her farm' – *Observer*

In My Wildest Dreams Leslie Thomas

The autobiography of Leslie Thomas, author of *The Magic Army* and *The Dearest and the Best*. From Barnardo boy to original virgin soldier, from apprentice journalist to famous novelist, it is an amazing story. 'Hugely enjoyable' – *Daily Express*

The Winning Streak Walter Goldsmith and David Clutterbuck

Marks and Spencer, Saatchi and Saatchi, United Biscuits, GEC ... The UK's top companies reveal their formulas for success, in an important and stimulating book that no British manager can afford to ignore.

A Turn in the South V. S. Naipaul

'A supremely interesting, even poetic glimpse of a part of America foreigners either neglect or patronize' – *Guardian*. 'An extraordinary panorama' – *Daily Telegraph*. 'A fine book by a fine man, and one to be read with great enjoyment: a book of style, sagacity and wit' – *Sunday Times*

Family Susan Hill

'This chronicle of the author's struggles to produce a second child reads like an account of a passionate love affair ... Perhaps the most remarkable thing about this book ... is how exciting it is. Harder to put down than most fiction' – Ruth Rendell

PENGUIN HEALTH

Audrey Eyton's F-Plus   Audrey Eyton

'Your short cut to the most sensational diet of the century' – *Daily Express*

Baby and Child   Penelope Leach

A beautifully illustrated and comprehensive handbook on the first five years of life. 'It stands head and shoulders above anything else available at the moment' – Mary Kenny in the *Spectator*

Woman's Experience of Sex   Sheila Kitzinger

Fully illustrated with photographs and line drawings, this book explores the riches of women's sexuality at every stage of life. 'A book which any mother could confidently pass on to her daughter – and her partner too' – *Sunday Times*

A Guide to Common Illnesses   Dr Ruth Lever

The complete, up-to-date guide to common complaints and their treatment, from causes and symptoms to cures, explaining both orthodox and complementary approaches.

Living with Alzheimer's Disease and Similar Conditions
Dr Gordon Wilcock

This complete and compassionate self-help guide is designed for families and carers (professional or otherwise) faced with the 'living bereavement' of dementia. With clear information and personal case histories, Dr Wilcock explains the brain's ageing process and shows how to cope with the physical and behavioural problems resulting from dementia.

Living with Stress   Cary L. Cooper, Rachel D. Cooper and Lynn H. Eaker

Stress leads to more stress, and the authors of this helpful book show why low levels of stress are desirable and how best we can achieve them in today's world. Looking at those most vulnerable, they demonstrate ways of breaking the vicious circle that can ruin lives.

PENGUIN HEALTH

Living with Asthma and Hay Fever   John Donaldson

For the first time, there are now medicines that can prevent asthma attacks from taking place. Based on up-to-date research, this book shows how the majority of sufferers can beat asthma and hay fever and lead full and active lives.

Anorexia Nervosa   R. L. Palmer

Lucid and sympathetic guidance for those who suffer from this disturbing illness, and for their families and professional helpers, given with a clarity and compassion that will make anorexia more understandable and consequently less frightening for everyone involved.

Medicines: A Guide for Everybody   Peter Parish

This sixth edition of a comprehensive survey of all the medicines available over the counter or on prescription offers clear guidance for the ordinary reader as well as invaluable information for those involved in health care.

Pregnancy and Childbirth   Sheila Kitzinger

A complete and up-to-date guide to physical and emotional preparation for pregnancy – a must for all prospective parents.

Miscarriage   Ann Oakley, Ann McPherson and Helen Roberts

One million women worldwide become pregnant every day. At least half of these pregnancies end in miscarriage or stillbirth. But each miscarriage is the loss of a potential baby, and that loss can be painful to adjust to. Here is sympathetic support and up-to-date information on one of the commonest areas of women's reproductive experience.

The Parents' A to Z   Penelope Leach

For anyone with children of 6 months, 6 years or 16 years, this guide to all the little problems involved in their health, growth and happiness will prove reassuring and helpful.

FOR THE BEST IN PAPERBACKS, LOOK FOR THE

PENGUIN HEALTH

Fighting Food   Marilyn Lawrence and Mira Dana

Fighting Food explains how society, the media and the family contribute to the suppression of women's needs which can result in a range of serious eating disorders. The authors also clarify the three main kinds – anorexia, bulimia and compulsive eating – demonstrating the links between them and discussing the best methods of treatment.

Medicine   The Self-Help Guide
Professor Michael Orme and Dr Susanna Grahame-Jones

A new kind of home doctor – with an entirely new approach. With a unique emphasis on self-management, *Medicine* takes an *active* approach to drugs, showing how to maximize their benefits, speed up recovery and minimize dosages through self-help and non-drug alternatives.

Defeating Depression   Tony Lake

Counselling, medication and the support of friends can all provide invaluable help in relieving depression. But if we are to combat it once and for all we must face up to perhaps painful truths about our past and take the first steps forward that can eventually transform our lives. This lucid and sensitive book shows us how.

Freedom and Choice in Childbirth   Sheila Kitzinger

Undogmatic, honest and compassionate, Sheila Kitzinger's book raises searching questions about the kind of care offered to the pregnant woman – and will help her make decisions and communicate effectively about the kind of birth experience she desires.

Care of the Dying   Richard Lamerton

It is never true that 'nothing more can be done' for the dying. This book shows us how to face death without pain, with humanity, with dignity and in peace.

FOR THE BEST IN PAPERBACKS, LOOK FOR THE

PENGUIN HEALTH

Healing Nutrients Patrick Quillin

A guide to using the vitamins and minerals contained in everyday foods to fight off disease and promote well-being: to prevent common ailments, cure some of the more destructive diseases, reduce the intensity of others, augment conventional treatment and speed up healing.

Meditation for Everybody Louis Proto

Meditation is liberation from stress, anxiety and depression. This lucid and readable book by the author of *Self-Healing* describes a variety of meditative practices. From simple breathing exercises to more advanced techniques, there is something here to suit everybody's needs.

The AIDS Handbook Carl Miller

Covering the full range of medical, personal and social consequences of the outbreak of AIDS, *The AIDS Handbook* is a powerful challenge to the idea that there is nothing we can do about this major health crisis. It cuts through the confusion to outline practical steps for everyone concerned about their own health or that of others.

Safe Shopping, Safe Cooking, Safe Eating Dr Richard Lacey

With listeria, salmonella and 'mad cow disease' hitting the headlines, many of our assumptions about the safety of everyday foods have been overturned. Here Dr Richard Lacey – the top microbiologist who made listeria a household word – tells you *everything* you need to know about food safety.

Not On Your Own Sally Burningham
The MIND Guide to Mental Health

Cutting through the jargon and confusion surrounding the subject of mental health to provide clear explanations and useful information, *Not On Your Own* will enable those with problems – as well as their friends and relatives – to make the best use of available help or find their own ways to cope.

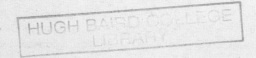